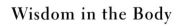

Wisdom in the Body

I wish many medical students will be given the opportunity to read Michael Kern's book. They will learn that they must develop their finger sensitivity. They will realise that their hands have a healing power.
Dr Michel Odent, obstetrician, pioneer of natural childbirth, founder of the Primal Health Research Centre, author of *Birthing Normally* and *The Scientification of Love*

Craniosacral therapy has always had an ambiguous relationship with osteopathy and 'cranial osteopathy' in particular. Michael Kern certainly acknowledges craniosacral's roots in osteopathy, but also makes the case for craniosacral therapy as a discrete discipline. Whichever way one inclines, this is an elegant, eloquent and very 'human' exposition of the work. For the student anticipating training, it glowingly represents the philosophy and principles behind practice and quotes quite delightfully some of the wise men and women in the field, right back to A. T. Still. The thoughtfulness and integrity of the material reflect a sincere and dedicated teacher and practitioner who seems to revel in the celebration of this approach to healthcare in whichever guise we see it and whatever name we give it.
Robert Lever B.A., D.O., Mem. GOsC, senior lecturer
European School of Osteopathy, Maidstone, England

Michael Kern's book *Wisdom in the Body* is both beautifully articulate and inspiring. Written for the lay person and health practitioner alike, this volume is a useful guide to the Breath of Life model of craniosacral work. Within this model the sacred relationship between spirit and matter is not only pondered and explored but utilized with skill and reverence to facilitate the expression of our inherent health. Michael's book will also serve as a resource for cranial practitioners of all lineages by providing another viewpoint from which to enrich our work.
Avadham Larson, L.Ac., CSTD, Certified CranioSacral
Therapy Instructor, Upledger Institute

This book has been written with the backing of long-term experience and I trust that it will benefit many people.
Venerable Dr Trogawa Rinpoche, head of Chagpori
Tibetan Medical Institute, Darjeeling, India

Wisdom in the Body is an effort towards a comprehensive, 'biodynamic' understanding of life. It is daring in its attempt to draw together abstract and cosmological concepts on the one hand, with specific and practical anatomical and physiological guidelines on the other. Michael Kern's case accounts are both instructional and warm. Of particular significance is his attempt to bring in the concept and treatment of trauma, and important applications of the Craniosacral approach to health in pregnancy and childbirth. This book is for practitioners at most levels as well as lay persons wanting to learn about the field.
Peter A. Levine Ph.D, author of *Waking the Tiger – Healing Trauma*

This is a well-written, practical overview of craniosacral therapy, one of the safest and most effective techniques for improving health that I have found in my investigations of treatments I did not learn in medical school. I now refer many patients to it and wish that more practitioners like Michael Kern were available.
Dr Andrew Weil, author of *Natural Health, Natural Healing, Spontaneous Healing* and *The Marriage of the Sun and Moon*

WISDOM IN THE BODY

The craniosacral approach to essential health

MICHAEL KERN

D.O., R.C.S.T., M.I.Cr.A., N.D.

Thorsons

Thorsons
An Imprint of HarperCollins*Publishers*
77–85 Fulham Palace Road,
Hammersmith, London W6 8JB

The Thorsons website address is: www.thorsons.com

Published by Thorsons 2001

10 9 8 7 6 5 4 3 2 1

© Michael Kern 2001

Michael Kern asserts the moral right to
be identified as the author of this work

A catalogue record for this book
is available from the British Library

ISBN 0 7225 3708 5

Text illustrations by PCA

Printed and bound in Great Britain by
Scotprint, Haddington, East Lothian

CONTENTS

ACKNOWLEDGEMENTS

With sincere thanks and acknowledgements to Franklyn Sills, who has helped to synthesize many of the ideas in this book. In appreciation of the depth and breadth of his vision, his generosity of spirit and his profound contribution to craniosacral work.

With deep gratitude to H. H. Gyalwang Drukpa for his tremendous gift of presence, boundless compassion and guidance.

Sincere thanks to Katherine Ukleja, Scott Zamurut, Mij Ferrett and Colin Perrow for their valuable insights and editorial contributions.

In memory of Ethel Blake, my grandmother, for her wisdom, encouragement and cheesecake.

For Sandrine Blanc, in gratitude for her wholehearted kindness and unselfish support during the writing of this book.

For Doreen, my mother, for all her love and support.

For Candice, whose love and good sense simply touch my soul.

PERMISSIONS

Quotes have been reproduced with kind permission from the following:

American Academy of Osteopathy, *Diagnostic Touch: Its Principles and Application* (Dr Rollin Becker D.O.; 1963 Yearbook)

—, *Diagnostic Touch: Its Principles and Application, Part 2* (Dr Rollin Becker D.O.; 1964 Yearbook)

—, *Diagnostic Touch: Its Principles and Application, Part 3* (Dr Rollin Becker D.O.; 1964 Yearbook)

—, *Diagnostic Touch: Its Principles and Application, Part 4* (Dr Rollin Becker D.O.; 1965 Yearbook)

—, *The Collected Papers of Viola Frymann* (Viola Frymann D.O., 1998)

—, *The Biological Basis for the Osteopathic Concept* (Dr I. M. Korr; 1960 Yearbook)

—, *Growth and Nutrition of the Body with Special Reference to the Head* (Dr A. G. Cathie; 1962 Yearbook)

Dr James Jealous D.O., *Around the Edges* (1996)

—, *Healing and the Natural World*; interview with Dr Jealous, 1997

Dr Harold Magoun Jr. D.O., F.A.A.O., F.C.A., *Osteopathy in the Cranial Field* (Harold Magoun D.O.; 1st edn; Sutherland Cranial Teaching Foundation, 1951)

—, *Osteopathy in the Cranial Field* (Harold Magoun D.O.; 3rd edn; Sutherland Cranial Teaching Foundation, 1976)

Dr Michael Shea Ph.D., R.C.S.T., *Somatic Cranial Work* (Shea Educational Group Inc., 1997)

Franklyn Sills M.A., R.C.S.T., *Craniosacral Biodynamics* (draft version), (North Atlantic Books, 2001)

Dr John Upledger D.O., O.M.M., in *Craniosacral Therapy* (John Upledger and Jon Vredevoogd; Eastland Press, 1983)

—, *Craniosacral Therapy 2, Beyond the Dura* (Eastland Press, 1987)

—, *Your Inner Physician and You* (North Atlantic Books, 1991)

—, *The Brain Is Born* (North Atlantic Books, 1996)

Cartoons have been reproduced with kind permission from:

Gerry Mooney, Dobbs Ferry, NY: *The Nervous System* (Figure 5.3) and *Animal Magnetism* (Figure 8.3).
Biff, London: *Craniosacral Therapists in Love* (Figure 7.1). Text revised by Michael Kern.

LIST OF ILLUSTRATIONS

FOREWORD

Franklyn Sills, M.A., R.C.S.T.

Health is universal. It is an expression of universal creativity. We live in a constantly creative universe. Each moment is a moment of creation. Our human system is an expression of this constant, moment-to-moment creation. Creation unfolds its intentions via the *Breath of Life*. The Breath of Life is a term used by Dr William Garner Sutherland to denote the intentions and actions of a universal Creative Intelligence at work. This mysterious Intelligence which we might call God or the divine, manifests its creative principle from the moment of conception until the day we die. This is expressed within the embryo as cellular motion and development.

Dr Sutherland maintained that the Breath of Life generates a *biodynamic potency* within the fluids of the body. This is an ordering force which orchestrates the form and function of the human body–mind. It is this biodynamic potency which maintains the original intention of a human being as an inherent blueprint of health, one which has an active physiological function. The potency of the Breath of Life maintains the health of every cell and tissue, and allows them to function in specific ways. It is within this process that organization is sustained and the experiences of life are centred and compensated for. The unfolding of the human system is thus a living biodynamic process in which the Breath of Life is constantly manifesting its creative intentions.

In this book, Michael Kern D.O. presents an approach of working within the craniosacral field which attempts to introduce and outline a biodynamic perspective within a clinical context. This is not an easy task, yet an introductory text is sorely needed. This viewpoint represents a paradigm shift from the concept of a *primary respiratory mechanism*, which expresses a mechanistic rhythmic impulse, to a dynamic system of tidal unfoldments which express the ordering imperatives of the Breath of Life. A biodynamic perspective is one in which the primacy of the Breath of Life is perceived and understood. It is one in which the action of the Breath of Life and the forces it generates are the focus for therapeutic work.

In the original cranial concept, the primary respiratory mechanism is outlined as a grouping of anatomical and physiological functions and parts which express a primary and subtle respiratory motion. It is composed of:

1 the inherent fluctuation of cerebrospinal fluid
2 the inherent motility of the brain and spinal cord
3 the mobility of reciprocal tension membranes
4 the articular mobility of the cranial bones and
5 the involuntary mobility of the sacrum between the iliac bones of the pelvis.

The perceptual shift to the primacy of the Breath of Life as the system's motivating and organizing factor is the foundation of a biodynamic understanding of the human system. Within this viewpoint, the human system is seen to organize as a unified field around the imperative of the Breath of Life. Thus, the concept of a primary respiratory mechanism, composed of tissue and fluid elements, shifts in emphasis to a wider system that expresses the primary respiratory function of the Breath of Life. Hence, the *primary respiratory mechanism* (P.R.M.) becomes the *primary respiratory system* (P.R.S.). This includes:

- the Dynamic Stillness at the heart of all motion
- the potency of the Breath of Life *per se*, which is called the Long Tide. This is a bioelectrical matrix organized around the primal midline of the body
- the organizing and integrating function of the potency of the Breath of Life within the fluids of the body
- the organization of the fluid and tissue systems to the imperative of the Breath of Life and its blueprint
- the expression of primary respiratory motion, in cycles of inhalation and exhalation, involving tissues, fluids and potency as a unit of function.

I have known Michael for many years now and he is a consummate clinician and experienced teacher. He is well placed to attempt to introduce concepts which are not easy to describe to a wider public. In the chapters which follow, Michael unfolds these concepts in a clear way from his own understanding and clinical practice. Again, this is not an easy task as the observations we make are always filtered through our personal perceptual processes and current use of words and terminology. I feel that Michael has done an admirable job here. In the end, the journey is to experience and explore these phenomena for ourselves, both inwardly and in relationship. This book is an important contribution to the field and I hope it will be widely read.

Franklyn Sills, Devon, England, January 2001

INTRODUCTION

My own story with craniosacral work began over 20 years ago, when as a disaffected college drop-out I first went for treatment. I was at a crossroads which seemed so big that I froze with fear. What was I going to do with my life? A tiredness had come over me which carried on for months. I felt a constant tightness in my head and struggled to drag myself out of bed each day. My family doctor told me that I had probably picked up a 'bug', but I left there feeling that he really didn't know what was happening. Around the same time, some close friends were enthusiastically singing the praises of a nearby craniosacral practitioner, so in despair I called for an appointment. I turned up for treatment with no idea of what to expect.

The thing that I most remember about those first appointments was how I felt heard. This was not because of any verbal reassurance or a sympathetic ear (although I'm sure that helped), but because I had never been touched like that before. My therapist put his hands on my head, hardly making contact, and waited there in silence. I had never experienced such a light and yet penetrating touch, or been in such close and yet spacious contact with another person. Within that contact it was as if the whole of me was being held: mind, body and heart.

Furthermore, this was not just a passive process, as I could sense a powerful re-organization taking place inside me. There was a clear and dynamic communication going on between the practitioner's hands and my body. His hand contacts had a precision and appropriateness, as if some primal part of me was being acknowledged. Slowly, slowly I began to notice that there was something else apart from my own confusion and the tightness my poor body had been carrying. I began to be aware of a depth of presence and healing, and started to let go.

With the help of craniosacral treatments, the pressure in my head lifted, my energy returned and I began to take on a new lease of life. I wanted to understand what happened and how it worked, so I started to take lots of courses, studying various forms of holistic medicine. I was hooked! After apprenticing with some highly-skilled and supportive teachers, I set up in practice. However, I soon reached another point when I didn't know what step to take next. Should I enrol on a lengthy osteopathic training and make a full commitment to this work? I decided to take some thinking time and travel along the west coast of America. One evening, just south of San Francisco, as my money was running out and the heaviness of indecision was looming, I went to a Chinese restaurant. At the end of the meal the waiter brought some tea and a fortune cookie. When I opened the cookie, the words which were enclosed leaped out at me: *'You will best succeed in a profession dedicated to the service of humanity!'* Prophetic intervention or not, it seemed enough to confirm my wish to study osteopathy, and so I returned to England to start the process of enrolment.

To my relief and surprise, and despite the reams of academic study and rote learning necessary to get through exams, I truly enjoyed going back to college. I became more deeply intrigued by the healing power of nature and the inexorable wisdom of the body. It was in osteopathy school that my explorations into craniosacral work began, and it has kept my interest ever since. A few years later, I started to teach craniosacral skills to osteopathic students and other health-care professionals, and have found that attempting to communicate this work to others has been a great excuse to further my own understanding.

This book has formed out of these years of treatment, learning, practice and teaching. My intention here is to present an outline of the craniosacral approach which can serve as a useful resource for the layman who wishes to dig a little deeper into 'how things work'. I hope that it will also be of value to craniosacral therapy students and other practitioners.

I hope to acquaint the reader to the fundamental principles of craniosacral work, looking at its developments from the initial insights of its founder, Dr William Garner Sutherland, to the present day. In this process, the layers of physiological functioning which essentially effect our health will be considered, in order to appreciate how we can work with ailments at the level of their origins. This book is not intended as an instruction manual, but as a guide to natural laws of healing and how they are applied in craniosacral work. Through these pages I hope the reader will grasp the immense potential of this approach to reconnect us to our source of health.

Over recent years craniosacral work has become one of the fastest-growing natural therapies. Increasingly, people have been coming for treatment because of their experiences at a grass-roots level. Patients of all ages and with a wide variety of conditions have been finding improvements in their health. Yet why these results occur has remained very much a point of debate. This is perhaps because, on the surface at least, nothing much seems to be happening during the treatment process. Unfortunately, many of the propositions that have been put forward take only a partial view of how we function. Any view which fragments us into our constituent parts, and in the process loses sight of the wider picture, tends to lead to confusion.

In this book, a *biodynamic* approach to craniosacral work is presented[1] – that is, one which acknowledges the inherent life-force in the body and our intrinsic wholeness. In our materialistic, mechanistic age, we often lose sight of the fact that we are more than just a collection of tissues, bones and fluids, as we seek to find explanations in physical terms only. Yet the acknowledgement of a *vital force* is at the heart of the craniosacral concept and was deeply appreciated by Dr Sutherland. He called it the *Breath of Life* and considered it to be the fundamental principle which maintains order and balance in the body.

The biodynamic approach has been further developed by practitioners such as Rollin Becker, James Jealous and Franklyn Sills. This book also includes insights from practitioners in related fields such as conventional allopathic medicine, physics, the spiritual traditions, psychotherapy and other therapy forms. These can all add to our understanding and perspective about how we function.

I'm aware that there is a lot of jargon which can creep into explanations of craniosacral work. However, the fact is that as human beings we are multi-faceted and complex. Some of the concepts in craniosacral work can be difficult to describe in words, as they are largely experiential and subjective. Consequently, I apologize if any ambiguity remains, but hope that the reader feels encouraged to investigate with their own experience what is being described. As the old saying goes, 'An ounce of practice is worth a ton of theory.'

While the use of some jargon is unavoidable, I have tried to stay with the languaging outlined by the founders of this approach, with the intention of encouraging consistency. In many cultures it is said that if we call something by its true name, then we can understand its nature.[2] Furthermore, craniosacral therapy is an approach which is firmly grounded in the anatomy of the body. This is where much of the power and efficacy of the work comes from. Consequently, many anatomical terms are used, but these have been kept to a minimum in order to make this book as accessible to the lay reader as possible.

I hope that nobody is put off by my consistent use of the male pronoun when referring to a practitioner. This does not imply any sexism, nor that highly skilled female craniosacral practitioners are not in abundance. In fact, women are often more able to develop the palpatory and perceptual skills required for craniosacral work. As the English language doesn't have any neutral pronouns, it seems more natural to stick to describing things from my own experience. Where the experiences of patients are described, although names have been changed, their true gender has been kept.

For me, this whole arena of work has been a journey of discovery. Each new patient who comes into the clinic is a teacher, if I listen to the unique story intelligently manifesting in their body. If this innate intelligence is appreciated, living skills rather than theories or techniques can be employed to support it. Craniosacral work is basically simple in its application: it is about how we can listen to the wisdom which is at our core, and help it to restore motion and health in our lives.

By contacting the core levels of health, the craniosacral approach is a gentle and powerful tool for the relief of suffering. It is an exploration into the essence of healing, one which has the potential to lead us to the deepest roots of our being.

Michael Kern, March 2001

1

THE HISTORY AND DEVELOPMENT OF CRANIOSACRAL WORK

Worms will not eat living wood where the vital sap is flowing; rust will not hinder the opening of a gate when the hinges are used each day. Movement gives health and life. Stagnation brings disease and death.

PROVERB IN TRADITIONAL CHINESE MEDICINE

BEGINNINGS

*My belief is in the blood and flesh as being wiser than the intellect. The
body-unconscious is where life bubbles up in us. It is how we know that we
are alive, alive to the depths of our souls and in touch somewhere with the
vivid reaches of the cosmos.*

D. H. LAWRENCE

Around the start of the 20th century, a final-year student of osteopathy, William Garner
Sutherland, was examining a set of disarticulated bones of a human skull in his college laboratory. Like other students of his time, Sutherland had been taught that adult cranial
bones do not move because their sutures (joints) become fused. However, he noted that he
was holding in his hands adult bones which had become easily separated from each other.

Like the gills of a fish

While examining the bevel-shaped sutures of a sphenoid and temporal bone (see Figure 1.1),
Sutherland had an insight which changed the course of his life. He described how a remarkable thought struck him like a blinding flash of light.[1] He realized that the sutures of the
bones he was holding resembled the gills of a fish and were designed for a respiratory
motion. He didn't understand where this idea came from, nor its true significance, but it
echoed through his mind.[2]

William Sutherland set out to try to prove to himself that cranial bones do not move, just
as he had been taught. As a true experimental scientist, he reasoned that if cranial bones
did move and that if this movement could be prevented, it should be possible to experience the effect. So he designed a kind of helmet made of linen bandages and leather straps
which could be tightened in various positions, thus preventing any potential cranial
motion from occurring.

Cranial movement

Experimenting on his own head, he tightened the straps, first in one direction and then in
another. Within a short period of time he started to experience headaches and digestive
upsets. This response was not what he was expecting, so he decided to continue his research
to find out more. Some of his experiments with the 'helmet' led to quite severe symptoms of
cranial tightness, headaches, sickness and disorientation. Of particular interest was that when

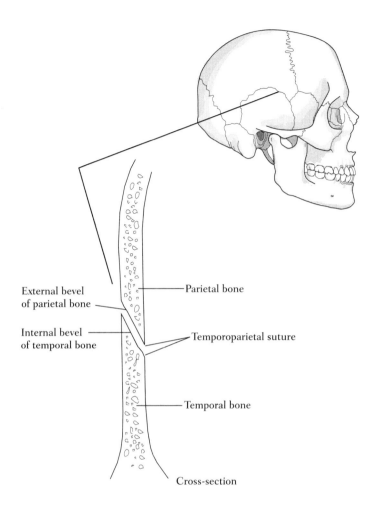

External bevel
of parietal bone

Internal bevel
of temporal bone

Parietal bone

Temporoparietal suture

Temporal bone

Cross-section

Figure 1.1: Bevel-shaped suture between temporal and parietal bones

the helmet straps were tightened in certain other positions, it produced a sense of great relief and an improvement in cranial circulation.[3]

After many months of pulling and restricting his cranial bones in different positions with these varying results, Dr Sutherland eventually stopped this research, having convinced himself that adult cranial bones do, in fact, move. Furthermore, the surprising responses that he felt in his own body had shown him that cranial movement must have some important physiological function. Sutherland spent the remaining 50 years of his life exploring the significance of this motion.

Historical acceptance

Although most Western countries did not recognize cranial motion, this possibility was not new to other cultures. There are various Oriental systems of medicine such as acupuncture and Ayurveda which have long appreciated the subtle movements which occur throughout the body, caused by the flow of our vital force or life-energy. This has also been traditionally taught in Russian physiology. Interestingly, anatomists in Italy in the early 1900s were already teaching that adult cranial sutures do not fully fuse, but continue to permit small degrees of motion throughout life.[4]

Cranial manipulation has been practised in India for centuries, and was also developed by the ancient Egyptians and members of the Paracus culture in Peru (2000 BC to 200 AD).[5] Furthermore, in the 18th century the philosopher and scientist Emmanuel Swedenborg described a rhythmic motion of the brain, stating that it moves with regular cycles of expansion and contraction.[6]

Tissue breathing

From an early stage, Dr Sutherland understood that he was exploring an involuntary system of 'breathing' in the tissues, important for the maintenance of their health. At a fundamental level, it is this property to express motion that distinguishes living tissues from those which are dead. Dr Sutherland perceived that all cells of the body need to express a rhythmic 'breathing' in order for them to function to their optimal ability. Much of his research was carried out by combining a profound knowledge of anatomy along with an acute tactile sense. He started to realize that these subtle respiratory movements can be palpated by sensitive hands. He also discovered that this motion provided a wealth of clinical information.

An interconnected system

Dr Sutherland recognized that the motion of cranial bones is connected to other tissues with which they are closely associated. The membrane system, which is continuous with cranial bones along their inner surfaces, is an integral part of this phenomenon. Significantly, Dr Sutherland also found that the central nervous system, and the cerebrospinal fluid which bathes it, have a rhythmic motion. The sacrum, too, is part of this interdependent system. Thus, there is an important infrastructure of fluids and tissues at the core of the body which express an interrelated subtle rhythmic motion.

As Dr Sutherland dug deeper into the origins of these rhythms, he realized that there are no external muscular agencies which could be responsible. He concluded that this motion is produced by the body's inherent life-force itself, which he called the *Breath of Life*.[7]

THE BREATH OF LIFE

Think of yourself as an electric battery. Electricity seems to have the power
to explode or distribute oxygen, from which we receive the vitalizing
benefits. When it plays freely all through your system, you feel well.
Shut it off in one place and congestion results.[8]
DR A. T. STILL

The inherent life-force of the body, the Breath of Life, was seen by Dr Sutherland to be the animator or spark behind these involuntary rhythms.[9] Alluding to the source of this phenomenon, other practitioners have referred to it as 'the soul's breath in the body'. The Breath of Life is considered to carry a subtle yet powerful 'potency' or force, which produces subtle rhythms as it is transmitted around the body.[10] Dr Sutherland realized that the cerebrospinal fluid has a significant role in expressing and distributing the potency of the Breath of Life. As potency is taken up by the cerebrospinal fluid, it generates a tide-like motion which is described as its *longitudinal fluctuation*. This motion has great importance in carrying the Breath of Life throughout the body and, as long as it is expressed, health will follow.

Expressions of health

The potency of the Breath of Life has remarkable properties for maintaining health and balance. An essential blueprint for health is carried in this potency, which acts as a basic ordering principle at a cellular level. This integrates the physiological functioning of all the body systems.

Dr Sutherland believed that the potency of the Breath of Life carries a basic Intelligence (which he spelled with a capital 'I'), and realized that this intrinsic force could be employed by the practitioner for promoting health.[11]

A similar concept is found in many traditional systems of medicine, where the main focus for healing is also placed on encouraging a balanced distribution of the body's vital force.[12]

The presence of full and balanced rhythms produced by the Breath of Life signifies a healthy system. As long as these rhythms are expressed naturally, the body's essential ordering principle is harmoniously distributed. Therefore, this rhythmic motion is primarily an *expression of health*. Its existence ensures the distribution of the ordering principle of the Breath of Life, and its restriction can have far-reaching consequences.

This brings us to two basic tenets of craniosacral work:

1 Life expresses itself as motion.
2 There is a clear relationship between motion and health.

Dr Harold Magoun D.O., a student and colleague of Dr Sutherland, described the intelligent action of the Breath of Life in the following way:

> *All life is manifested in energy or motion. Without motion, in some degree, there can only be death. Furthermore, motion is essential to function. But that motion must be intelligent and purposeful for the living organism to successfully compete with its environment. Hence that motion must be guided and directed by a Supreme Being. There must be a channelling of the Universal Intelligence down to the individual cell or organism. Otherwise all would be chaos. What is the Supreme Intelligence? How does the channelling take place? No one knows for sure. The fact remains that the existence of such is a positive and irrefutable fact which is emphasized by the world's greatest scientists.*[13]

Primary respiratory motion

Dr Sutherland named the system of tissues and fluids at the core of the body which express a subtle rhythmic motion the *primary respiratory mechanism* (see Figure 1.2). As these tissues are not under voluntary muscular control, they are also sometimes referred to as *the involuntary mechanism* (or I.V.M.). Dr Sutherland used the term 'primary' because this motion underlies all others. It is the manifestation of the life-stream itself. Every cell expresses this *primary respiratory motion* throughout its life. Significantly, many different symptoms and pathologies which involve both body and mind are related to disturbances of primary respiratory motion.

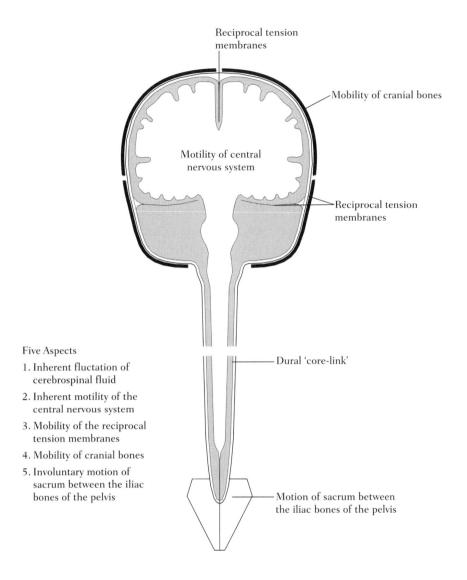

Reciprocal tension
membranes

Mobility of cranial bones

Motility of central
nervous system

Reciprocal tension
membranes

Five Aspects

1. Inherent fluctuation of
   cerebrospinal fluid

2. Inherent motility of the
   central nervous system

3. Mobility of the reciprocal
   tension membranes

4. Mobility of cranial bones

5. Involuntary motion of
   sacrum between the iliac
   bones of the pelvis

Dural 'core-link'

Motion of sacrum between
the iliac bones of the pelvis

Figure 1.2: The primary respiratory mechanism

There are, of course, other vital rhythmic motions in the body such as the heartbeat and lung respiratory breathing. Although necessary for the maintenance of life, these are considered 'secondary' motions because they are not the root cause of the body's expression of life. Without the Breath of Life there would be no other motion. Lung respiration or the breathing of air is therefore sometimes called *secondary respiration*.[14]

This fact was proved to Dr Sutherland early on in his development of this work. During the days of prohibition in America during the 1920s, he was staying at a cottage on the shores of Lake Erie. One day he heard a commotion outside, when a man who had been drinking far too much illegal liquor was being dragged out from the water. By the time Dr Sutherland reached the shore, the man was lying on the ground. His normal life signs (lung function and cardiovascular pulse) had ceased, and all attempts to resuscitate him had failed.

With some quick thinking, Dr Sutherland took hold of the sides of the man's head and encouraged a rocking motion of his temporal bones, in an attempt to stimulate primary respiratory motion.[15] This worked; within a few seconds the man's breathing and heartbeat started up again and he regained consciousness. This experience helped to affirm to Dr Sutherland the tremendous power of working directly with the Breath of Life.

Sustained by the Breath of Life

The importance of an underlying vital force for the maintenance of health has been demonstrated by many reliable accounts of seemingly magical feats performed by advanced practitioners of yoga. Some of these feats include being buried alive for up to seven days, with no access to air, water, food or light. Amazingly, it seems that these advanced yogis are able to sustain their bodies by going deep into meditation and being conscious of the fact that their lung breathing is not the main thing keeping them alive. It seems that they are able to suspend many of the 'secondary' physiological functions of the body, but still preserve the 'primary' expression of the Breath of Life. Their survival depends on their ability to maintain this fundamental life-giving principle.

The expression of the Breath of Life at a cellular level is a fundamental necessity for good health. If the rhythmic expressions of the Breath of Life become congested or restricted, then the body's basic ordering principle is impeded and health is compromised. The main intention of craniosacral work is to encourage these rhythmic expressions of health. This is done by gently facilitating a restoration of primary respiratory motion in places where inertia has developed.

SPREAD OF THE WORK

Nature heals, the doctor nurses.
PARACELCUS

Dr Sutherland developed various therapeutic approaches to harness the intrinsic power of the Breath of Life and help resolve any restrictions to primary respiratory motion. He began to teach this work to other osteopaths from about the 1930s, and tirelessly continued to do so until his death in 1954. Challenging, as it did, some of the closely held beliefs among practitioners of the time, his work was at first largely rejected by the mainstream osteopathic profession. However, his clinical results in a wide range of cases were impressive and he began to attract a small band of osteopathic colleagues who wished to study with him.

In the 1940s the first osteopathic school in America started a post-graduate course called 'Osteopathy in the Cranial Field' under the tutelage of Dr Sutherland. Soon after, others followed. This new branch of practice became known as *cranial osteopathy*. As the reputation of cranial osteopathy began to spread, Dr Sutherland trained more teachers to meet the demand. The most notable of these early teachers were Drs Viola Frymann, Edna Lay, Howard Lippincott, Anne Wales, Chester Handy and Rollin Becker.

However, even today many osteopathic colleges do not teach this work on their basic courses, and so it is often studied as an option at post-graduate level. Consequently there are many practising osteopaths who do not use this approach. Nevertheless, in the last few years post-graduate training courses for practising osteopaths have become widely available.

Dr John Upledger

In the mid-1970s Dr John Upledger was the first practitioner to teach some of these therapeutic skills to people who were not osteopathically trained. Dr Upledger had become drawn to exploring primary respiratory motion after an incident that occurred while he was assisting during a spinal surgical operation. He was asked to hold aside a part of the dural membrane system which enfolds the spine, while the surgeon attempted to remove a calcium growth. To his embarrassment, Dr Upledger was unable to keep a firm hold on the membrane, as it kept rhythmically moving under his fingers.[16] He took a post-graduate course in cranial osteopathy and then set out on his own path of clinical research. Over the years, Dr Upledger has developed some clear and practical perspectives about the impact of trauma on the primary respiratory mechanism, and a combined mind–body approach for working with traumatic experience, called *somato-emotional release*. He has done a great deal to popularize craniosacral work around the world.

When Dr Upledger began to teach non-osteopaths, he encountered great opposition from many in the profession who believed that the foundation of a full osteopathic training is necessary to practise the craniosacral approach. Many osteopaths are still of this opinion, and it continues to be a cause of much debate and argument. However, many also believe that this work can provide an integrated approach to health care in its own right and need not remain within the sole domain of osteopathic practice. Nevertheless, one thing is for sure: a good foundation in anatomy, physiology and medical diagnosis is necessary in order to apply craniosacral work with safety and competency. It also takes time and proper training to develop the necessary skills. It is an unfortunate fact that in recent years there are many people who have set up in practice with only minimal training.

Cranial osteopathy and craniosacral therapy

It was Dr Upledger who coined the term 'craniosacral therapy' when he started to teach to a wider group of students. Dr Upledger wanted to differentiate the therapeutic approaches he had developed and, furthermore, the title 'cranial osteopath' could not be used by those new practitioners who were not osteopathically trained.

One question I'm frequently asked is, 'What is the difference between cranial osteopathy and craniosacral therapy?' Although Dr Upledger states that these two modalities are different,[17] the differences are not always so obvious. They both emerge from the same roots and have much common ground, yet different branches have developed. A variety of therapeutic skills are now commonly used by both osteopaths and non-osteopathic practitioners of this work, so neither cranial osteopathy nor craniosacral therapy can be accurately defined by just one approach. However, in practice, craniosacral therapists often work more directly with the emotional and psychological aspects of disease. Aware that I'm running the gauntlet of professional politics, in this book I use the term 'craniosacral' to include the whole body of work from the early pioneering cranial osteopaths to more recent developments in the field.

Craniosacral biodynamics

In the biodynamic view of craniosacral work, which is predominantly referred to in this book, an emphasis is placed on the inherent healing potency of the Breath of Life. In this approach, the functioning of the body is considered to be arranged in relationship to this essential organizing force.[18] This has practical ramifications for the way in which diagnosis and treatment are carried out, as will be explored a little later. This way of working also has a direct link to the pioneering insights of Dr Sutherland. It's interesting to note that during the latter years of his life, Dr Sutherland focused his attention more and more on working directly with the potency of the Breath of Life as a therapeutic medium.[19] He saw that if the expression of this vital force can be facilitated, then health is consequently restored. Dr Rollin Becker, Dr James Jealous and Franklyn Sills have each added valuable insights into the operation of these natural laws which govern our health.

In the last 15 years there has been a huge increase of interest in craniosacral work. It is now taught and practised in many countries around the world. As this work is largely unregulated by law, professional associations have now been set up in many of these countries. At the back of this book there is a Resource Guide of training schools and professional organizations which keep registers of qualified practitioners.

2

THE CRANIOSACRAL
CONCEPT

The same stream of life that runs through my

veins night

and day runs through the world and dances in

rhythmic measures.

It is the same life that shoots in joy through

the dust

of the earth in numberless blades of grass

and breaks

into tumultuous waves of leaves and flowers.

It is the same life that is rocked in the

ocean-cradle

of life and death, in ebb and flow.[1]

RABINDRANATH TAGORE

THE THREE TIDES

Life manifests itself like a development of fluctuations; up and down,
hunger, sleep, waking up, feeling like working, feeling like resting, etc.
When we start feeling that behind these fluctuations there is something
immutable, we stop being perturbed.[2]
ITSUO TSUDA

The craniosacral concept focuses on how we function in mind, body and spirit, on very subtle layers of physiology. At the basis of this concept is an understanding about the workings of the Breath of Life and the critical role played by its rhythmic motion in carrying our essential forces of order and balance.

In this chapter we will explore some of the different aspects of the integrated physiological system of the Breath of Life, often referred to as the *primary respiratory system*. We will also draw comparisons from the world of modern physics.

Life as motion

As we noted, life is expressed as motion. All living cells demonstrate this basic truth. They breathe with the Breath of Life, which vitalizes them and maintains the numerous physiological functions necessary for survival.

As the Breath of Life is expressed in the body a series of tide-like rhythms are generated, producing subtle movements which can be felt in the tissues. This motion initially arises at the core of the body and involves the central nervous system, the cerebrospinal fluid, and surrounding membranes and bones. The manifestation of these rhythms in the tissues of the body denotes the effective distribution of the Breath of Life and is indicative of healthy function.

The cyclical rhythms of the Breath of Life have two phases of motion. These can be described as a 'breathing in' and a 'breathing out'. These phases are called *primary inhalation* and *primary exhalation*.

During the inhalation phase there is a subtle motion which rises upwards and at the same time expands from side to side, orientated around the midline of the body (see Figure 2.1).

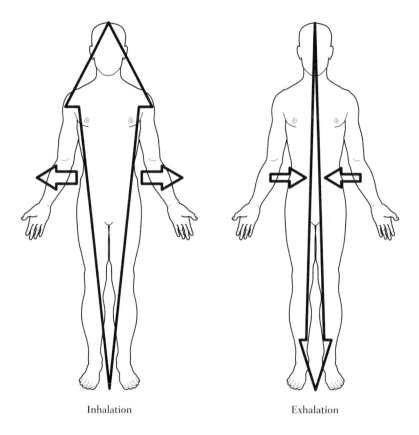

Inhalation   Exhalation

Figure 2.1: Primary inhalation and exhalation

During the exhalation phase the opposite occurs: a motion which recedes down towards the lower part of the body and narrows from side to side.

These movements manifest in all parts of the body, producing rhythms which have been scientifically measured and can be palpated by sensitive hands.

The combination of an inhalation and an exhalation phase constitutes one rhythmic *cycle*.

From the core of our being there are a succession of rhythms that emerge, creating a whole system of primary respiratory motion. There are three main rhythms which have been identified. These all express phases of inhalation and exhalation at a different rate, and are sometimes referred to as the 'three tides' (see Figure 2.2).

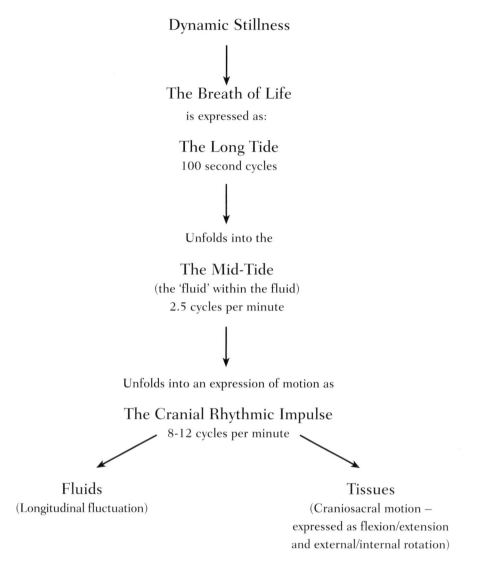

Figure 2.2: The primary respiratory system

Each of the three tides is a manifestation of a different level of functioning of the Breath of Life. Each one is enfolded in the others, producing rhythms within rhythms, known as:

- the cranial rhythmic impulse
- the mid-tide
- the long tide.

Cranial Rhythmic Impulse

As the Breath of Life is conveyed into the body, it sets up a very slight rocking motion of all fluids, bones, membranes and organs. Individual tissue structures behave like boats gently rocked on the surface of the ocean. This motion occurs at an average rate of between 8–12 cycles per minute and is called the *cranial rhythmic impulse* (C.R.I.). The cranial rhythmic impulse is considered to be the outermost (i.e. most superficial) unfoldment of the Breath of Life.

In optimal health all the tissues and fluids of the body express the cranial rhythmic impulse with balance and symmetry. The cerebrospinal fluid expresses this motion as a longitudinal fluctuation, rising up the body in inhalation and receding in exhalation.

Each tissue structure expresses a specific pattern of motion during these inhalation and exhalation phases. These patterns are described as either *flexion/extension* or *external/internal rotation*, and refer to how individual parts of the body move in their relationship to each other. This is commonly called *craniosacral motion*. The particular way each structure expresses its craniosacral motion will be described in more detail in the next chapter.

Research experiments

The cranial rhythmic impulse has been measured in numerous research experiments. In 1963, American osteopath Dr Viola Frymann clearly recorded these minute contractile and expansile movements at the cranium.[3] These experiments were the first in which a rhythmic motion not directly connected to either heartbeat or lung breathing was scientifically identified. Since that time, a growing number of investigators have been able to measure this phenomenon. In a later experiment (1978), recordings of pulse rate and lung breathing were taken, along with measurements from different regions of the head.[4] These recordings again clearly showed that the cranial rhythmic impulse is a distinct motion not directly related to heartbeat or lung respiration.

It must be emphasized that the movements produced by the cranial rhythmic impulse are minuscule. They are measured on a scale of *microns* (each micron is one-millionth of a metre). The greatest motion measured at the cranial bones is 40 microns, about half the thickness of a piece of paper.[5]

Drs John Upledger and Zvi Karni conducted experiments recording subtle movements at both the cranium and the sacrum. They used sensitive strain gauges and measured changes in the electrical potential of the skin.[6] Their instrumentation picked up changes in motion, which were simultaneously detected by manual palpation. These experiments affirmed the ability of the human hand to be sensitive to these small movements.

In another experiment, Dr Upledger and colleagues measured the cranial rhythmic impulse of patients in a coma or with chronic neurological disorders. Again, measurements were taken with strain gauges and checked by palpation. They found that these patients all exhibited a slowing down of the cranial rhythmic impulse to about a half of the normal level.[7] Upledger and Karni were also able to establish that these rhythmic movements are detectable all over the body.

Self-palpation

You may be able to feel these movements in your own head. To do this, find a comfortable and quiet place to sit. With a lightness of attention, place your hands on your head. Gently cup the sides of your head with your palms (see Figure 2.3). You may be more comfortable doing this leaning slightly forwards, with your elbows resting on your knees.

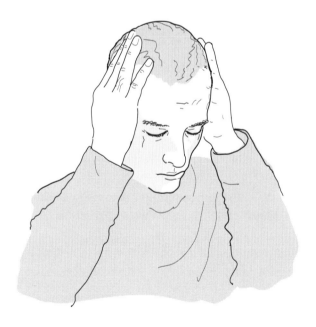

Figure 2.3: Self-palpation

First, become aware of your heartbeat. Then, notice your lung respiratory breathing. Then, see if you notice anything else. Place your attention into the tissues under your hands. See if you can perceive a very subtle motion slower than both your heartbeat and lung breathing. Try to feel this by placing your attention on what may be happening underneath these other two movements. Let your hands just float on your cranial bones, as if they were gently resting on corks floating on the tide. If you press too hard you will prevent the 'corks' from expressing their motion. Create some space inside yourself to allow any impressions come into your hands.

Do you notice a sense of welling up and receding of fluid in your hands, like the movement of a tide? This may be the longitudinal fluctuation of cerebrospinal fluid. Do you notice a widening and narrowing from side to side of the 'corks'? This may be the external and internal rotation of bones at the side of the head. You may also get a sense of the tissues' inner breathing, or motility.

Variable rates

The rate of the cranial rhythmic impulse (C.R.I.) is relatively stable if compared to the heartbeat or lung breathing, which easily fluctuate according to our circumstances. For example, the heart and lungs show dramatic changes in rate depending on whether we are in a state of rest or activity. They also vary in response to changes in our environment, or as a result of strong emotion. Although the heart and lungs adjust more obviously to changes in life circumstances, the rate of the C.R.I. nevertheless does vary. These variations tend to indicate changes in physiological function which occur at a deeper level.

The C.R.I. will often, for example, speed up in cases of acute illness and fever. In this way the ordering principle of the Breath of Life carried in these rhythms is made more available. The C.R.I. may also quicken in hyperactive or anxiety states. It tends to slow down in more chronic states of fatigue or depression, and also congestive conditions such as persistent headache or catarrh. Resistances held in the tissues of the body can also seriously affect the expression of the C.R.I.

What is significant is that the C.R.I. records how our essential health is being expressed, and the influence of any conditioning. This makes it an accurate barometer of mental, emotional and physiological patterns. Consequently its palpation may be used as a clear indicator of health and disease, involving both mind and body.

Origin of motion

There has been much debate in the craniosacral profession about what exactly causes these rhythmic impulses. Some practitioners believe they are generated in response to a cyclical production and reabsorption of cerebrospinal fluid (see next chapter). Others place an emphasis on the motion of the central nervous system. There is also a suggestion that the cranial rhythmic impulse (C.R.I.) is produced by involuntary muscle contraction, causing the delivery of a rhythmic movement to cranial bones and the central nervous system.[8] Still others believe the C.R.I. is produced by a combination of many different factors, including lung breathing and arterial pulsations. In the *entrainment theory* it is suggested that there is a pooling of various motions and pulsations produced by both patient and practitioner.[9] A coherent rhythm may be created as these pulsations harmonize together.

Clearly this is a subject where further research is still needed. None the less, there can be no doubt that this rhythmic motion is a real and palpable phenomenon. Whatever the particular mechanisms which produce or disseminate the C.R.I., there still remains the question of 'what moves these mechanisms?'

If we wish to investigate the actual origins of this motion, there is an overwhelming argument for acknowledging the crucial presence of an underlying vital force, the potency of the Breath of Life. I emphasize this point because it is frequently not included by those who take a more mechanistic approach.

To summarize: the outermost rhythmic expression of the Breath of Life is called the *cranial rhythmic impulse* (C.R.I.). The particular ways in which it manifests in the body is called *craniosacral motion*. It is here, with the C.R.I., that most people have their first experience of primary respiratory motion. It is also here that many therapists focus their work. However ... there are also deeper and slower rhythmic movements which underlie the C.R.I.

The Mid-Tide

In the course of clinical practice, many practitioners have become aware of tidal forces operating behind the cranial rhythmic impulse.[10,11,12] These deeper tides also have a rhythmic motion, and are considered by many to be the driving power that produces the C.R.I. Although these rhythms are somewhat more subtle, they can also be detected by palpation. The particular rhythm which directly underlies the C.R.I. is expressed at a slower rate, of approximately 2.5 cycles per minute. It is sometimes referred to as the *mid-tide*.[13]

The mid-tide is considered to carry the available bio-energy, or *biodynamic potency*, which vitalizes the body. It also expresses phases of inhalation and exhalation. In inhalation the mid-tide rises up the body and widens from side to side. In exhalation it recedes while narrowing from side to side. This motion is naturally orientated around the midline of the body.

The rate of the mid-tide is far less affected by our immediate conditions than the C.R.I. Its rate is consequently very stable.

Biodynamic potency

The biodynamic potency in the mid-tide is of great significance because it carries the essential ordering force of the Breath of Life. Therefore it has a profound ability to maintain physiological integration and balance at a core level. The potency of the mid-tide promotes health and healing in all tissues where it is able to manifest.

When the mid-tide is tuned in to, it is often experienced as a sense of unity and well-being which permeates the body, bringing a feeling of wholeness. It may be felt by settling into a state of stillness and taking a 'wide view' of ourselves (for more details, see Chapter 6). One patient described an experience of the mid-tide in his own body 'like slipping down a boat ramp and sliding *into* the water'.[14] In fact, accessing the mid-tide is like dropping beneath the surface of the ocean. It is like being in a submarine rather than a boat.

Inner breathing

As the mid-tide is expressed in tissues and fluids, it causes them to 'breathe' simultaneously at this slower rate. This inner breathing of tissues is called *motility*. All living structures express motility, including even seemingly hard and rigid ones like bones. Our usual perception of bone as a hard and lifeless substance is derived from the fact that only dead and dried specimens are usually examined. However, living bone is teeming with life. It contains a blood and nerve supply, a high percentage of fluid, and possesses a remarkable degree of flexibility for motion. When teaching this work, Dr Sutherland often implored his students to focus on what occurs in *living* tissues.[15]

As a result of the motility produced by the mid-tide, individual structures of the body are stimulated to express their craniosacral motion. As Dr Becker observes, 'The tissue elements, the muscles, ligaments, bony structures, the organ systems within their connective tissue envelopes, and their fluid contents, automatically go along for the ride as the bioenergy patterns unfold in their functioning.'[16]

Role of fluid

The fluid systems of the body play an important role in distributing our biodynamic potency. Fluid acts as the medium into which potency is rhythmically expressed at the rate of 2.5 cycles per minute. Potency becomes infused in the fluids, which irrigate the whole body and convey this vital force to all regions. Therefore an unrestricted motion of fluid within the body is critical for the dissemination of biodynamic potency and the maintenance of health.

The biodynamic potency of the Breath of Life has been described as 'the energy free to act within the fluids'.[17] This potency may be experienced as a kind of 'fluid within the fluid'.[18] A similar concept is found in Chinese medicine, where the fluids of the body are also considered to carry vital forces and a basic ordering principle. It's important to remember that *all* living tissues contain fluid which serves this function. In fact, each cell of the body can be likened to a tiny sac of fluid, in which its microscopic internal structures are 'floating'.

Spark in the motor

Since the early days of this work, craniosacral practitioners have particularly recognized the significant role of cerebrospinal fluid (C.S.F.) in carrying the potency of the Breath of Life. C.S.F. is the 'juice' which bathes the central nervous system. It is also the vehicle into which biodynamic potency is initially expressed in the body. C.S.F. can thus be seen as the principal link between the potency of the Breath of Life and its expression in the body.

The potency expressed within cerebrospinal fluid acts as the 'spark in the motor',[19] motivating the longitudinal fluctuation of fluid which occurs as part of the faster cranial rhythmic impulse. Dr Sutherland had a deep appreciation of this vital force carried in C.S.F., and considered it to be central to the workings of primary respiratory motion.[20] He described the potency of the Breath of Life as an 'invisible element' found within C.S.F. and the force which makes it move.[21] The remarkable properties of C.S.F. will be considered in more detail in the next chapter.

The Long Tide

Emerging from the ground of our being, the first stirring of the Breath of Life sets up a very deep and slow rhythmic impulse. This can also be palpated in the body as it rises/expands and recedes/narrows along the midline. This even slower rhythm is often referred to as the *long tide* and is a subtle radiance of the most essential qualities of the Breath of Life. The long tide is, in fact, the subtlest manifestation of our life-force. It underlies and supports all other activities in the body.[22]

Perceiving the long tide is like dropping down near to the ocean floor. The long tide directly underlies the mid-tide, serving as the force behind it. The other, faster rhythms are generated from the long tide, as the Breath of Life unfolds into its outer manifestations. Each rhythmic cycle of the long tide is expressed at a rate of about once every 100 seconds. It has a very light, airy quality as it permeates the body as our most essential life breath. This is sometimes experienced as a shimmering or a subtle electrical wind.

Deepest resource

In comparison to the faster tides, the long tide is not affected by the vagaries of day-to-day experiences and conditioning. It is an expression of a deeper and more subtle layer of functioning. This tide is very stable in its nature and rate, as it gently resonates and rhythmically permeates the body from the core of our being. At a profound level, it contains the knowledge to create healing. It is at the foundation of all regulatory functions of the body and, clinically, its emergence indicates a reconnection to our deepest resource of health.

GROUNDSWELL OF THE BREATH OF LIFE

And Lord God formed man of the dust of the ground, and breathed into
his nostrils the Breath of Life, and man became a living soul.[23]
GENESIS 2:7

Intrinsic stillness

From our deepest source, the Breath of Life is conveyed in the series of unfoldments described above as the 'three tides'. However, at our very core there is a state of pure, unfabricated being and stillness. This is the place of our deepest nature. This essential ground state is underneath all our individual traits, our personality and all our doing. It's like the ocean floor.

If we deeply quieten ourselves, dropping our attention into the source from which all our activities emerge, we may catch glimpses of this state of intrinsic stillness. At this level there is no duality, no subject and no object. Many spiritual traditions refer to this realm as our fundamental and primordial state. In Buddhist texts it is described as having qualities of emptiness and luminosity. This state of stillness is contained at the basis of all forms, and the full potential of all forms is to be found within it. It is this reality that the Buddha described when he taught, 'Form is emptiness, emptiness is form, form does not differ from emptiness, emptiness does not differ from form.'[24]

Life emerges

All expressions of life emerge out of stillness. As our being manifests into becoming, the Breath of Life starts to express itself as a succession of motions. This sets up the different tidal rhythms of the primary respiratory system. This process can be compared to how a wheel turns. At the hub of the wheel there is stillness. However, as you move towards the periphery, motion takes place at a faster rate (see Figure 2.4).

Essentially what is being described here is a coming about of our individuation, an emergence into form. This process of creation is happening every single moment of our lives, and is organized around the creative intention of the Breath of Life. It was described by Dr Sutherland as a *groundswell*.[25] The groundswell of the Breath of Life refers to the stirring of life as it manifests from the ground of our being.

This groundswell motion arises with a centrifugal force (a movement outwards), followed by a centripedal return to the source (a movement inwards). These centrifugal and centripedal forces rhythmically arise from and return to the source as the most basic expression of life (see Figure 2.5). These forces may be perceived as spiral movements of energy, like the coiling and uncoiling of a spring in constant motion.[26]

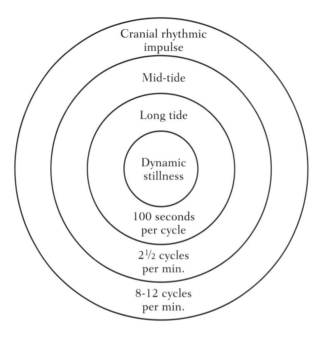

Figure 2.4: The three tides emerging out of stillness

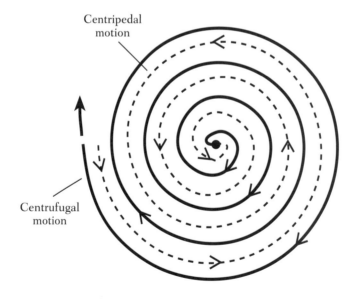

Figure 2.5: The groundswell of the Breath of Life

Genesis

The body is in a constant state of repair, regulation and regeneration. At each moment, the vitalizing forces of the Breath of Life hold the whole process together, bringing order and integration. As Dr James Jealous describes,

> *The Breath of Life comes into the body. We can sense various rhythms*
> *that are created from it, and we can perceive that process taking place ...*
> *We can actually perceive the Breath of Life come into the body, come*
> *into the midline, and from the midline, generate different forms of*
> *rhythms in the bioelectrical field, fluids and tissue. Essentially what's*
> *happening is genesis. It never stops. Moment to moment we are*
> *building new form and function.*[27]

Dr Jealous is describing an extraordinary thing: a direct perception of the Breath of Life coming into the body. This is a moment of creation in which our form and all our physiological activities are being generated by the expression of the Breath of Life.

Transmutation

Many craniosacral practitioners regard the primary respiratory system as a kind of transformer, which steps down the powerful energies of the basic life-breath into the physical body. From their source of stillness, the emergence of each rhythm signifies a further condensation into form. This can be compared to how electrical power is brought into a city on 44,000-volt power lines, and then stepped down to 110 volts so that it can be used.[28] Dr Sutherland called this process a *transmutation*.[29]

Change of state

Transmutation refers to a change of state. Like ice can turn to water and then to steam, a transmutation is a becoming of something new, a kind of 'shape-shifting'.[30]

Each emerging unfoldment of the Breath of Life is a change of state. In this process each new state is formed out of the one which underlies it. From the ground of dynamic stillness, motion arises. This is a transmutation which is expressed as the long tide. Then the mid-tide is generated, a rhythmic motion taken up within the fluids of the body. This unfolds into the faster longitudinal fluctuation of cerebrospinal fluid and the craniosacral motion of tissues.

THE HOLOGRAPHIC PRINCIPLE

*Relativity and, even more important, quantum mechanics have strongly
suggested (though not yet proved) that the world cannot be analysed into
separate and independently existing parts. Moreover, each part somehow
involves all the others: contains them or enfolds them.*[31]

DR DAVID BOHM

The human organism can be seen as a unified system of function in which the whole is contained in every part. This same idea is found in a variety of health care systems such as acupuncture, Ayurvedic medicine, polarity therapy, reflexology and iridology. In these therapies, individual parts of the body such as the pulse on the wrist, the texture of the tongue, zones on the feet or regions of the eye are used to reveal information about the functioning of the whole system.

This principle is also illustrated by the genetic building blocks contained in every cell, called DNA. Each cell contains coiled strands of DNA which hold the inherited information of the entire body. Each cell contains information of the whole, enabling the creation of compatible new cells with the same genetic imprint.

Holographic model

The different tidal rhythms produced by the Breath of Life make up a whole system of interrelated motion, the primary respiratory system. Each layer of the primary respiratory system is contained within the other, creating a unified field of activity. Therefore, each part of this system is interconnected and has access to the whole.

In the holographic view of the universe, each and every physical form is considered to be interconnected in this way. This concept was pioneered by researchers such as Stanford neurosurgeon Dr Karl Pribram and the renowned quantum physicist Dr David Bohm.

What is a hologram?

The behaviour of light illustrates how the holographic principle works. A hologram is a special type of three-dimensional projected image, produced by a beam of pure laser light. A laser beam is passed through a prism, which then splits it into two separate branches (see Figure 2.6[i]). One branch of the laser beam is aimed at an object being photographed, and

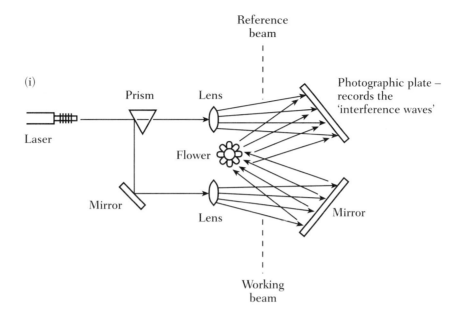

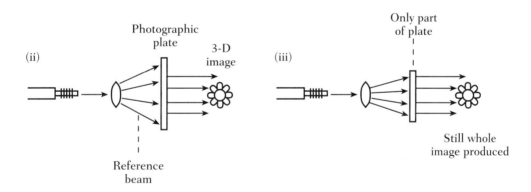

Figure 2.6: The formation of a hologram[32]

as a result the object is reflected back onto a photographic plate or film. The other branch of the split laser beam is aimed directly at the photographic plate.

Let's say that the object being photographed is a flower. The beam of light projected onto the flower is called the *working beam*. When the working beam meets the flower, it splits up into various wave forms like the scattered ripples produced in flowing water when it encounters a rock. In this way the working beam becomes diverted or 'conditioned' by encountering the flower. Some of the ripples of light bouncing off the flower are reflected onto the photographic plate.

The other branch of laser light from the prism, however, maintains its coherence. It is still pure unadulterated laser light, unconditioned by meeting any object.[33] This beam is called the *reference beam*. It is also reflected onto the photographic plate.

Where the light waves from both the working beam and the reference beam meet, *interference patterns* are produced. Where these interference patterns reach the photographic plate, they are recorded on film which stores a three-dimensional image of the hologram. If you then shine another beam of pure laser light through the photographic plate, a complete three-dimensional image of the flower is produced in the space behind it (see Figure 2.6[ii]).

Whole in the part

Let's imagine that, after recording the image of the flower, the photographic plate is accidentally dropped and shatters into many small pieces. One would probably think that at least a part of the image would be lost. However, each broken piece is still able to produce an image of the whole flower (see Figure 2.6[iii]). This is because each individual part of the plate contains the whole picture in an encoded form. One of the key features of a hologram is that information of the whole is contained within each part. In other words, each part has access to the whole.[34]

Reference beam

Let's imagine that the reference beam becomes blocked while the image is being made, and only the 'ripples' created when the working beam encounters the flower reach the photographic plate. When you then attempt to produce a holographic image, no clear or coherent picture will be generated, only chaotic patterns.[35] However, if some of the 'ripples' from the working beam become blocked, an image will still be produced. So, in the production of a hologram the reference beam is fundamentally necessary to maintain the order and integrity of the encoded image. Without the coherence provided by the reference beam, only chaotic images are produced.

An organism can be viewed as a kind of holographic system in which everything is intrinsically connected. Furthermore, the reference beam of a hologram is akin to the essential ordering principle of the Breath of Life, which maintains the integrity and coherence of the body. If the Breath of Life becomes blocked or restricted, then disorder or chaos results and coherence is lost. One of the main intentions of craniosacral work is to reconnect parts which have become chaotic to the 'reference beam' of the Breath of Life.[36]

Holographic memory

One of the great mysteries which has puzzled neuro-scientists is how the brain stores memory. Even though various parts of the brain may be damaged or even removed by surgery, memory can still remain intact. This shows that there is not any one particular physical location in the brain which carries out the function of memory. It seems that memory is enfolded throughout the whole brain.

Dr Karl Pribram proposes that the brain operates in many ways like a hologram.[37] He suggests that memory is stored in a similar way to how holographic images are stored on a photographic plate. If this is the case, it would explain how a specific memory does not have a location but is distributed throughout the brain.[38] In the holographic model, each part of the brain contains information relating to the whole and therefore has access to every other part.

Holograms require a source of coherent light. Recent research indicates, in fact, that the brain has the ability to communicate and process information via pathways of light. This is in addition to the linear communication that takes place through nerve pathways. Evidence has been found that brain cells may emit coherent light in organized waves.[39] These light waves provide the ideal medium in which memory could be holographically distributed. Some researchers suggest that cerebrospinal fluid is the vehicle which carries this light.[40] In fact, tiny particles of energy, bio-photons, which have the capability of emitting light, have been found in the life fluids of all living organisms.[41]

Implicate and explicate order

Dr David Bohm proposed that there is a unifying principle which holographically links the whole of creation. He surmised that although all forms in creation appear to be separate on the outside, they are, in fact, connected by an underlying implicit order. Dr Bohm referred to a 'holographic universe' which has two aspects: an inner *implicate realm* and an outer *explicate realm* (see Figure 2.7).

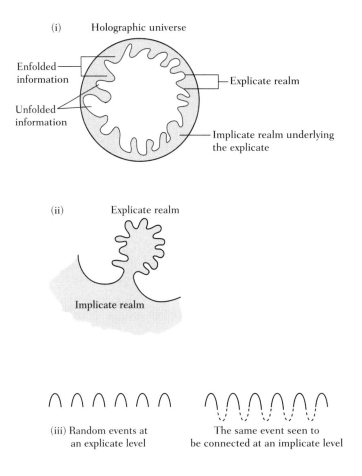

(i)   Holographic universe

Enfolded information

Explicate realm

Unfolded information

Implicate realm underlying the explicate

(ii)   Explicate realm

Implicate realm

(iii) Random events at an explicate level

The same event seen to be connected at an implicate level

Figure 2.7: Implicate and explicate realms[42]

The implicate realm is a domain of undivided wholeness, which is at the basis of all forms. The explicate realm is the domain where things appear (at least on the surface) to be separate. This is what we can see with our eyes. However, the implicate realm of wholeness is always contained within each explicate part. Franklyn Sills notes, 'What may at first appear to be unrelated random occurrences, may actually be completely interrelated at an implicate level.'[43]

These proposals fit very well with Dr Sutherland's view of the primary respiratory system. In the craniosacral concept, the tidal rhythms of the Breath of Life emerge from an implicate realm of dynamic stillness. Within each emerging state, all others are enfolded – rather like a set of Russian dolls. In the primary respiratory system, there are interpenetrating rhythms within rhythms, derived from a unified field. Each rhythmic unfoldment is a particular expression of an enfolded universal principle.

Realm of unity

According to the holographic view, everything in life is connected to everything else, and everything is contained in everything else. It is even thought that the whole universe is holographically contained within every single atom.[44] Each atom can be seen as an individual little universe, in which electrons revolve around one another just like the sun and planets in the outer universe.[45]

The presence of an intrinsic realm of unity is acknowledged in many spiritual traditions, as well as in modern quantum physics. For example, both Christianity and Judaism refer to God or the 'divine' as an indivisible universal principle. The whole Eastern philosophy is founded on the principle that there is an essential unification of matter and experience. Buddhists refer to this underlying state as *shunyata* – our true, enfolded, unmanifested nature. The quintessential religious experience of oneness and unity described by mystics may be a clear experience of this implicate and universal ground.[46]

This view suggests that the essential wholeness at the ground of our being can be intrinsically found within any single part. It is by reconnecting to the implicate realm that our greatest potential can be accessed and most fundamental healing take place. Going back to this source of wholeness, it may be possible to wipe the slate clean and start over again.

ORIGINAL MATRIX

Health can be defined as the emergence of Originality. The Originality expresses a complete balance of both structure and function as intentionalized in the creation of a human being.[47]
DR JAMES JEALOUS

Embryological imperative

From the very moment of conception, the body forms around a precise and primary design. As the first cells of the body start to divide, they somehow know how to create a human being

... as opposed to something else! An extraordinary degree of order and intelligence is apparent in this process. However, it has been found that at this early stage there are no genetic mechanisms capable of promoting such organized development. According to the leading embryologists Blechschmidt and Gasser, the ordering and organization of our early development does not occur as a result of genetics operating through our DNA. As they state, 'Hereditary factors are an important, but not the only condition for the process of differentiation ... The genes themselves do not perform the differentiation process.'[48]

Apparently, genetic influences do not begin to fully operate until about six weeks *after* conception.[49] Therefore, an important question arises: what provides the coherence of our early growth? Drs Blechschmidt and Gasser propose that there is an ordering principle that brings about this organization, operating through the fluids of the body. Significantly, this is the same conclusion that Dr Sutherland came to when considering the role that fluid plays in carrying the intrinsic ordering principle of the Breath of Life.

Essential blueprint

The Breath of Life carries an essential blueprint for health, called the *Original Matrix* by Dr James Jealous. This blueprint is a deep and unwavering ordering principle intrinsically distributed around the body in the tidal rhythms of primary respiratory motion. The original matrix has also been described as an *original intention*, because it is present at the very beginning of life as the cells of the embryo begin to form and differentiate.[50] However, this same embryological imperative continues throughout life, in each moment of creation. The rhythms of the Breath of Life continuously deliver an intrinsic order into the fluids, and thus into each cell of the body. The various tissue and fluid systems of the body form around this essential blueprint and are maintained by it, until the time of death. As long as there is life, this ordering principle is never lost.[51] Franklyn Sills concludes,

> *In healing work this is a critical point to understand. No matter how desperate the situation, the information of the whole, its inherent ordering principle, or blueprint, is still available in each part. The blueprint of health is thus present in each part and is still available if it can be accessed.*[52]

Facilitating order and health

Because the original matrix is distributed in the cycles of primary respiratory motion, the ability of cells to express the Breath of Life has important consequences for their health. At a fundamental level, primary respiratory motion maintains each cell's order and integrity. The aim of craniosacral treatment is to facilitate the expression of the original matrix in tissues which have become disordered and affected by pathology. By encouraging the manifestation of the Breath of Life at a cellular level, the craniosacral therapist acts as a facilitator of this essential blueprint for health. According to Dr Jealous,

> It is the permeation of the Breath of Life into disorientated tissues that re-establishes the Original Matrix. The Original Matrix is a form that is carried through the potency of the Breath of Life around which the molecular and cellular world will organise itself into the Original pattern set forth by the Master Mechanic.[53]

Sarah's story

Sarah's case illustrates how the re-emergence of the original matrix may be experienced. Sarah had come for craniosacral treatment because of a serious and persistent low back problem. Her doctor had recommended surgery to remove one of her spinal discs, but Sarah was reluctant to go ahead with this and was looking for an alternative. When tuning in to her primary respiratory system from the feet, the intrinsic wisdom in her body began to take over. What follows is her own personal description.

Sarah started to feel a slow wave move through her body. This wave began at her feet, moved through her legs, up into her lower back and then into the disc which was causing trouble. As this wave permeated the area of her low back, she literally felt a rearranging of the tissues around the disc. The wave continued up her spine, but then got stuck at the occipital bone at the base of her skull. She started to feel an intense pain there. She then had a strong image come into her mind, 'Oh, my god! I remember coming off a motorbike and biting the back of a bus!' Sarah had had an accident a few years previously, when she had landed face-down in an open-backed bus, knocking out a few teeth. She then remembered that after this accident she had had to undergo lots of dental work, and flashbacks of this time started to come back to her. She next felt the wave move from the back of her head to her face, and then back down through her body. At this point the pain and the images associated with her accident all remarkably disappeared. Sarah then exclaimed, 'My body now feels how it was intended to!'[54]

Inviolable wisdom

The subtle rhythms produced by the Breath of Life are considered to be the primary self-regulating and self-healing forces in the body. Dr Sutherland described that the potency of the Breath of Life carries an inviolable and unadulterated wisdom, beyond the relatively meagre intelligence of human ideas and concepts.[55] This potency carries our original matrix of health. Therefore the balanced expression of primary respiratory motion ensures a constant distribution of inherent health to all cells of the body. In the words of Dr Rollin Becker,

> *It provides the physiological evidence of health within the whole body physiology as well as evidence of less than health for any area of dysfunction. It can be used as a diagnostic tool as well as being a tool for treatment, and it is a manifestation of life within the patient that the physician can use in his service to restore health to the patient.*[56]

3

THE PRIMARY RESPIRATORY MECHANISM

Know your anatomy and your physiology, but
when you get your hands on a patient's body,
never forget that a living soul dwells therein.

DR A. T. STILL

CRANIOSACRAL MOTION

The rhythmic, involuntary mobility of the tissues and
fluids and the various tides are all totally integrated
with each other and with the body as a unit.[1]
DR ROLLIN BECKER

One thing that becomes clear when considering the physiological functioning of the body is the remarkable order that underlies its complexity. The systems of the body are guided by a wisdom which is actually a manifestation of our own basic nature. This inherent, intelligent force of integration and wholeness makes itself available through the rhythms of the Breath of Life.

In this chapter we will take a look at the key tissue and fluid systems at the core of the body which express primary respiratory motion. We will also look at the significance of these different tissues, and the particular ways that they impart the cranial rhythmic impulse.

In order to get a sense of how these tissues function, it is necessary to have an understanding of their anatomy. Therefore, a review of major anatomical features is also included in this chapter.

Craniosacral rhythm

All the bones, membranes, fluids and organs of the body express the cranial rhythmic impulse (C.R.I.) as a specific pattern of movement, their *craniosacral motion*. These are like individual wave-forms which ride on deeper tidal forces.[2] By comparison, the slower mid-tide is expressed in the fluids (and consequently in *all* tissues) of the body as a dynamic and unified field of motion.[3]

The cyclical rhythms of craniosacral motion have the characteristic of *reciprocal tension*, a kind of tensile pushing and pulling that is produced in the tissues. This is expressed first as a movement one way, and then as a movement back. These tissue rhythms function at the average rate of between 8–12 cycles per minute. This motion is also sometimes called the *craniosacral rhythm*, or abbreviated to the *cranial rhythm*.

Mobility and motility

Each structure of the body expresses a rhythmic primary respiratory motion as both *mobility* and *motility*. 'Mobility' refers to the movement of a particular structure in relationship to another, for example at a joint or suture, or between different organs. In fact, each structure in the body expresses an individual pattern of craniosacral mobility. This kind of motion occurs solely as a function of the C.R.I.

'Motility' refers to the inner breathing of tissues, a motion that arises from within a particular structure. Motility occurs as the direct expression of the potency of the Breath of Life, which motivates and enlivens tissues from the inside. Motility is normally expressed in tissues as a welling up and expansion from side to side, followed by a narrowing.

It is thought that craniosacral mobility occurring between structures is essentially generated by their intrinsic motility.

Primary respiratory mechanism

After Dr Sutherland discovered the existence of motion involving cranial bones, he embarked on a path of enquiry which led him to dig deeper for further understanding.[4] He realized that there is a system of inter-related tissues at the core of the body, all of which play an important role in primary respiratory motion. These are the tissues and fluids in and around the dural membrane system, a continuous tissue infrastructure which surrounds the brain and spinal cord.

This inter-connecting system of tissues and fluids is referred to as the *primary respiratory mechanism* (see Figure 1.2, page 7). These tissues comprise the cerebrospinal fluid, the central nervous system, the membranes which surround the central nervous system, the cranial bones and the sacrum. These five core aspects are also sometimes called the *craniosacral system*. The physiological motion of these five aspects is considered to have important consequences for the whole body; many pathologies can be traced back to some disturbance in their function.

In health, all aspects of the primary respiratory mechanism operate in a harmonic relationship. Each part expresses its craniosacral motion in a specific way, but they function together as part of an integrated system.

The different aspects of the primary respiratory mechanism can be compared to the different instruments in an orchestra, which all play the same music but contribute in different ways to the overall 'sound', while the Breath of Life conducts the symphony.

Two phases

Craniosacral motion is rhythmically expressed in two phases. However, these two phases are described in different ways, according to which parts of the body are being referred to. The terms *inhalation* and *exhalation* are used to describe the craniosacral motion of the cerebrospinal fluid (C.S.F.) and the central nervous system. These rise and widen from side to side during the inhalation phase, and descend and narrow from side to side during the exhalation phase.

All the other structures of the body express their craniosacral motion in phases which are described as:

- *flexion* and *extension*
- *external* and *internal rotation*.

Flexion and extension refer to the motion of single midline structures. One example of such a midline structure is the occipital bone, centrally placed at the back of the head (see Figure 3.13, page 65).

External and internal rotation refer to the motion of all paired structures of the body. The two parietal bones 'capping' the top of the head, one on the left and one on the right, are examples of paired structures (see Figure 3.1).

Flexion of the midline structures and external rotation of the paired structures occur simultaneously during the inhalation phase of craniosacral motion. For example, while the central nervous system and C.S.F. are expressing inhalation, the occipital bone moves into flexion and the parietal bones move into external rotation.

Extension and internal rotation occur simultaneously during the exhalation phase.
To summarize, the craniosacral motion of different parts of the body is described as:

- Inhalation – central nervous system and fluids: ⎫ all occurring
- Flexion – midline structures: ⎬ at the
- External rotation – paired structures: ⎭ same time

38

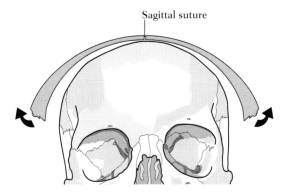

Inhalation - external rotation

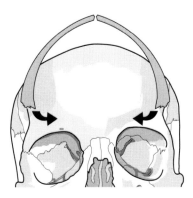

Exhalation - internal rotation

Figure 3.1: External and internal rotation of the parietal bones

- Exhalation – central nervous system and fluids: } all occurring
- Extension – midline structures: at the
- Internal rotation – paired structures: same time

FIVE CORE ASPECTS

The primary respiratory mechanism has been broken down into five
components for teaching purposes, but it remains one unit of function.[5]
DR ROLLIN BECKER

In this section we will explore the tissue and fluid systems which constitute the core elements of the primary respiratory mechanism. These pages contain quite a lot of information about some of the specific ways that primary respiratory motion is expressed in the body. To bring this information alive, see if you can sense how these tissues are organized in your own body. The corresponding diagrams may help you to picture clearly what is being written about. If you are unfamiliar with some of the anatomical terms which are being used, please refer to the Glossary at the back of the book.

The five principal aspects which constitute the primary respiratory mechanism play an important role in expressing the Breath of Life and regulating the balance of health. Although these tissues have great significance, primary respiratory motion is also a feature of the whole body. Therefore, we will also be considering how the body acts as a unit of integrated physiological function, and the particular ways that craniosacral motion is expressed by all fluids, connective tissues, bones, organs and muscles.

The five components at the core of the primary respiratory mechanism are:

1 the inherent fluctuation of cerebrospinal fluid (C.S.F.)
2 the inherent motility of the central nervous system
3 the mobility of the reciprocal tension membranes
4 the motion of cranial bones
5 the involuntary motion of the sacrum between the iliac bones of the pelvis.

1) The Inherent Fluctuation of Cerebrospinal Fluid

The inherent fluctuation of cerebrospinal fluid (C.S.F.) refers to its tide-like motion through the body, contained within the membranes which surround the central nervous system.

C.S.F. is a transparent, slightly yellowish fluid, produced by a process of filtration and secretion. This occurs within specialized tissues called *choroid plexi* (see Figure 3.2). These are cauliflower-shaped growths of blood vessels located in the fluid-filled cavities of the brain, the *ventricles*. The choroid plexi filter blood entering the brain, adding certain substances such as magnesium and chloride, while potassium and calcium are removed.[6] The choroid plexi also filter out any harmful materials which may be carried in the blood. Therefore, C.S.F. has a different chemical composition from blood, distinctly suited to maintain the delicate balance of the central nervous system, which it bathes. Approximately 150 ml of C.S.F. is contained in the cavities of the brain and spinal canal at any one time, and its total volume is replaced (i.e. produced and reabsorbed) every 3 to 4 hours.

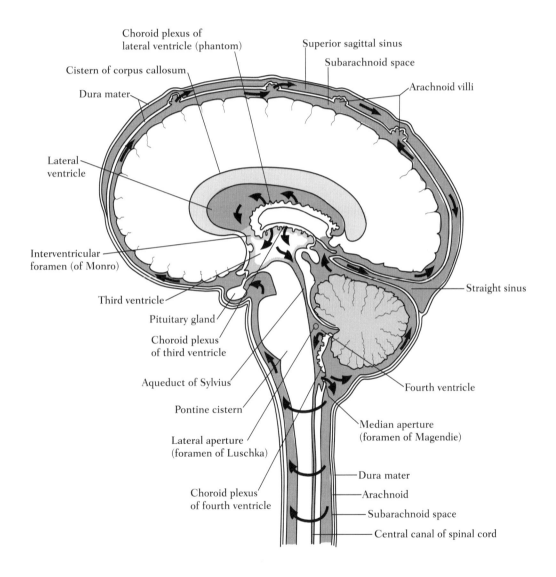

Figure 3.2: Circulation of cerebrospinal fluid

Circulation of C.S.F.

C.S.F. circulates around the central nervous system, before being reabsorbed back into the bloodstream. This reabsorption occurs via small projections – the *arachnoid villi* – which are located in the drainage channels of the head, called *venous sinuses* (see Figures 3.2 and 3.10, page 41 and page 58). The system of venous sinuses in the head connect with veins, which transport the reabsorbed C.S.F. back to the heart. However, radioactive tagging has also indicated that small amounts of C.S.F. escape from the spinal column through sheaths of connective tissue which surround the spinal nerves (see Figure 3.19, page 78).[7] The hollow collagen fibres within these connective tissues provide the medium through which C.S.F. can pass into the rest of the body.

Physiology of C.S.F.

C.S.F. provides essential nourishment for the central nervous system, helping it to maintain a consistent chemical balance, even when other conditions of the body are changing. All the critical functions which are mediated by the central nervous system are dependent upon the proper supply of this fluid. If the physiology of C.S.F. is disturbed, the functioning of the central nervous system can be affected, with vast ramifications for the health of the whole body.

Over 100 years ago, Dr A. T. Still, the visionary founder of osteopathy, paid particular attention to the properties of C.S.F. He wrote,

> *Cerebrospinal fluid is the highest known element that is contained in the
> human body and unless the brain furnishes this fluid in abundance a
> disabled condition of the body will remain. He who is able to reason will
> see that this great river of life must be tapped and the withering fields
> irrigated at once or the harvest of health be forever lost.*[8]

It is known that the nervous system degenerates if the choroid plexi (which produce C.S.F.) are removed.[9] Furthermore, there is also recent evidence that the choroid plexi tend to deteriorate in the elderly. This suggests that certain types of brain disorders, such as Alzheimer's disease, may be caused by an inadequate C.S.F. production.[10] Any deficiency in the production of C.S.F. will lead to malnutrition of the brain.

C.S.F. has a number of other crucial roles to play. Waste products are rinsed from the central nervous system by the steady flow and reabsorption of C.S.F. It provides 'water beds' for the protection of the brain, acting as a shock absorber and helping to maintain the shape of the brain.[11] C.S.F. also dampens the physical effects that the pulsation of arteries can have on the central nervous system.

If all the vital physiological functions of C.S.F. are considered, the importance of encouraging its proper flow and interchange can be appreciated. There seems to be much truth in the statement made by Dr Harold Magoun when he called C.S.F. 'a regulatory complex which transcends any and all other agencies throughout the body'.[12]

Inherent fluctuation

In addition to its circulation around the central nervous system, C.S.F. also has a tidal motion – described as an *inherent fluctuation*. The fluctuation is called 'inherent' because it moves due to a power found within itself, not because of any external force. The fluctuation of C.S.F. is a motion which ebbs and flows along the body in rhythmic cycles. Like the ocean tides this is a movement of the whole volume of fluid at the same time, rather than a current or a wave.

In many ways, the body displays similar properties to the planet on which we live. Dr Sutherland not only compared the rhythmic fluctuation of C.S.F. to the tide of the ocean, but also concluded that it is governed by the same great intelligence which governs the ocean tide ... and the motion of all the planets.[13] In Chinese medicine our connection to the natural world is well recognized. According to the Chinese system, C.S.F. is controlled by 'kidney energy' and the kidneys are governed by the moon. Therefore the moon, which governs the tides of the oceans, also governs the functioning of C.S.F. within the body.

The tidal motion of C.S.F. is also described as a *longitudinal fluctuation* because it moves up and down along the length of the body. As we noted, there are two phases to this longitudinal fluctuation, described as inhalation and exhalation. C.S.F. rises up the body in inhalation and recedes down the body in exhalation. In inhalation there is also a welling up of fluid from side to side, as it rises. In exhalation there is a side-to-side narrowing of the fluid. Whereas the ocean tide rolls onto the seashore twice a day, this fluctuating motion of C.S.F. in the body occurs on average about 10 times per minute.[14]

Pressurestat mechanism

Over the years there have been a number of theories which have attempted to explain how the longitudinal fluctuation of C.S.F. is initiated. Below is an outline of some descriptions commonly put forward, although none has been proven.

Some practitioners have suggested that this motion is generated by movements in the central nervous system.[15] Dr John Upledger proposes that it occurs due to the way C.S.F. is produced and reabsorbed. He describes a rhythmic build-up of C.S.F. controlled by a *pressurestat mechanism*. In this model, the membrane sac within which C.S.F. circulates is seen as a semi-enclosed hydraulic system. Pressure is maintained in this system because it contains only partial openings—i.e. the places at which C.S.F. is produced and reabsorbed.

Dr Upledger proposes that C.S.F. production at the choroid plexi is pulsatile.[16] He suggests that, normally, production goes on for about 3 seconds, then stops for about 3 seconds, and then repeats. He also suggests that reabsorption via the arachnoid villi is constant. In this way, an expansive rhythm is produced about every 6 seconds, or 10 cycles per minute. Dr Upledger surmises that there are sensitive nerve reflexes which are located in the sagittal suture between the two parietal bones at the top of the skull. As the hydraulic system fills with C.S.F., these nerve reflexes get stretched and send messages to the choroid plexi to stop producing C.S.F.

Ball valve mechanism

It has also been proposed that a *ball valve mechanism* may control the drainage of C.S.F.[17] The *straight sinus* is one of the main channels in the venous sinus system, helping to drain reabsorbed C.S.F. away from the head. A bundle of tissue composed of arachnoid villi has been identified at the entrance to this channel. It is thought that this tissue can become engorged with blood in rhythmic cycles, thus intermittently blocking the passage of fluid through the straight sinus. This mechanism may help to control the outflow of fluid from the head and rhythmically increase the pressure of C.S.F. within the system. This pressure increase may then affect the production of C.S.F. at the choroid plexi, which temporarily shuts off as a result. When the ball valve mechanism unblocks the straight sinus, pressure is reduced and C.S.F. production resumes.

However, recently I witnessed a spinal operation which for me casts doubt that either of the above mechanisms can explain how longitudinal fluctuation occurs. In this operation the surgeon was demonstrating a revolutionary technique of grafting some nerve tissue into a patient's spinal cord, which had been severed during an accident. When the membranes surrounding the spinal cord were opened, there was still a marked surge of C.S.F. about every 6 to 8 seconds, clearly visible as it rose up into the opening. If the pressurestat model or the ball valve mechanism were correct, then it would not have been possible for C.S.F. to continue its fluctuating motion once the spinal membranes were open, as this would have altered the pressure dynamics upon which these models are based. In my view it seems there is still no better explanation for this phenomenon than that originally proposed by Dr Sutherland: the motion of C.S.F. is an inherent fluctuation arising from a potency found within itself. No doubt this is a topic for further research!

Fluid drive

The potency behind C.S.F. motion produces what is sometimes described as the system's *fluid drive*. A strong fluid drive indicates a plentiful expression of the Breath of Life being taken up in C.S.F. This generates a more powerful surge and settling of its longitudinal fluctuation, and is indicative of a good availability of healing resources for the whole body. However, fluid drive may become diminished in states of chronic illness or exhaustion. Therefore, the quality of fluid drive is a useful baseline for the practitioner to establish in the assessment of a patient's condition. It can provide a wealth of clinical information about the body's state of constitutional health.

Highest known element

The pioneering cranial practitioners had a deep appreciation of the subtle yet powerful properties of C.S.F. Dr Sutherland realized the significant function carried out by this fluid early on in his investigations of primary respiratory motion. In addition to its physical properties, he perceived that C.S.F. provides an important connection between the potency of the Breath of Life and its expression in the body. C.S.F. is considered to be the initial recipient of the Breath of Life, playing an essential role in taking up and distributing its potency. This concurs with Dr Still's view that C.S.F. is the 'highest known element in the body'.[18] The basic ordering principle of the Breath of Life is carried around the body primarily within this fluid medium.

Carrier of potency

Dr Sutherland saw the biodynamic potency of the Breath of Life as a kind of 'fluid' which is carried within the C.S.F.[19] He often described the potency in the fluid as 'liquid light'.[20] Dr Magoun referred to this phenomenon as 'an electrical potential'.[21] Consequently, C.S.F. has been compared to the battery fluid of the body, which can be recharged with potency.[22] It is this charge of potency which provides C.S.F. with remarkable healing properties. Dr Sutherland had no doubt that C.S.F. is the key element in the craniosacral concept.[23] The free and unrestricted movement of C.S.F. is a major factor in promoting health.

Other practitioners have also recognized the exceptional functions carried out by C.S.F. Dr Randolph Stone, an osteopath who developed the practice of Polarity Therapy, described C.S.F. as 'a storage field and conveyor of ultrasonic and light energies. It bathes the spinal cord and is a reservoir for these finer essences ... Through this neuter essence, mind functions in and through matter as the light of intelligence.'[24]

C.S.F. is the primary meeting point between the Breath of Life and the body. It is a junction between the physical and the spiritual; an essence which conducts the life-principle through the body, like the life-giving sap in a tree.[25] According to nuclear physicist Dr R. T. Lustig,

> *Through nuclear physics we are just catching a glimpse of what cerebrospinal fluid really is ... a vital mechanism which affords powerful influences upon human physiology ... A cold analysis of research in kindred fields ... points unmistakably to the buried potential in the cerebrospinal fluid ... With the opening of the atomic age we are getting a better perspective of energy, its sources and conversions ... Sutherland's work ... puts him on record as having recognized at an early date the interchangeability of energy and matter as it relates to biology.*[26]

This view of C.S.F. is not only compatible with much modern research, but is also alluded to in many historical sources. A respected 18th-century anatomist, Burton, referred to the brain ventricles (which are filled with C.S.F.) as 'the receptacles of the spirits'.[27] C.S.F. has been called the 'brain dew' and referred to as 'the nectar of life', 'the divine fluid', and 'tears of the sky of God'. Can C.S.F. also be the allegorical 'ambrosia' of ancient Greece, the all-sustaining beverage of the gods who resided on Mount Olympus (i.e. the brain)? Or perhaps it is the divine nectar called *Soma* referred to in the ancient Vedas of India?[28] Dr Magoun asserts, 'As long as life exists this highest known element is the abiding place of that mysterious spark which cannot be explained but is none the less present.'[29]

Peter's case

Peter was a film producer who had been experiencing sharp headaches, which often started after any kind of exertion. He was also exhausted, perhaps due to work stress and having recently moved house. He was starting to become very concerned because his symptoms were not improving and extensive medical tests had not been able to reveal any cause for his condition. When he lay down on the treatment table, I tuned in to how primary respiratory motion was being expressed in his body.

I put my hands on Peter's head and my first impression was that the strength of potency in his system was very low. This was revealed by the fact that the quality of his 'fluid drive' was weak. Furthermore, there was an area of tension at the base of his skull, where it appeared that the longitudinal fluctuation of C.S.F. was getting congested.

The first aim of treatment was to try to build up Peter's constitutional resources. This was done by encouraging what are called 'stillpoints' in his body. These are periods of settling and stillness of the cranial rhythmic impulse, which allow for deep physiological rest. This enables the 'battery fluid' of the body (i.e. C.S.F.) to recharge with potency (see also Chapter 7, Stillpoints). I then started to work with the area of tension at the base of Peter's head, by making subtle suggestions of 'decompression' through my hands. This region can have an important effect on the drainage of fluid from the head and, if restricted, may cause the congestion of C.S.F. During Peter's third treatment this tension completely resolved, leading to an immediate improvement in the longitudinal fluctuation of his C.S.F. and the strength of its fluid drive. Peter remarked it was 'like someone switched a light on inside my head!' After this his energy increased and headaches disappeared.

2) The Inherent Motility of the Central Nervous System

The soft and gelatinous tissues of the brain, together with the spinal cord, express their primary respiratory motion in the form of a motility, occurring at the rate of about 8–12 cycles per minute. A number of researchers have confirmed the presence of a rhythmic motility of nerve tissue occurring at this rate.[30] In 1987 medical researchers Feinberg and Mark demonstrated the motion of the human brain using magnetic resonance imaging, although they linked this motion to the pulse of the circulatory system.[31] As another researcher commented, the brain is 'vibrantly alive ... incessantly active ... dynamic ... highly mobile ... able to move forwards, backwards, sideways, circumduct and to rotate'.[32]

Embryological development

Generally speaking, the patterns of growth which tissues follow when they are being formed in the embryo determines the pattern of their craniosacral motion throughout life. In this way, the central nervous system expresses its motility along the axis of its embryological development.

At about the third week after conception, a bundle of rapidly developing cells called the embryonic disc starts to fold in on itself at the midline (see Figure 3.3). As the sides of the embryonic disc heap up and join in the middle, a hollow structure called the *neural tube* is formed. The brain and spinal cord develop as outgrowths around this tube (see Figure 3.4). The neural tube then elongates, bulges outwards, and by the fifth week starts to fold in on itself at the top. By the end of the fifth week the formation of the specific structures of the brain has begun (see Figure 3.4[ii]). As the tissues around these folds grow out in a curling pattern, the brain is formed (see Figures 3.4[iii and iv] and 3.5).

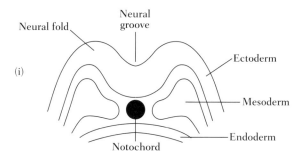

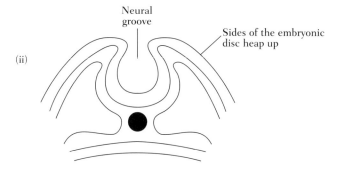

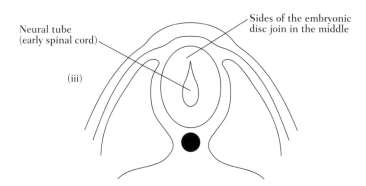

Figure 3.3: Formation of the neural tube (cross-section)[33]

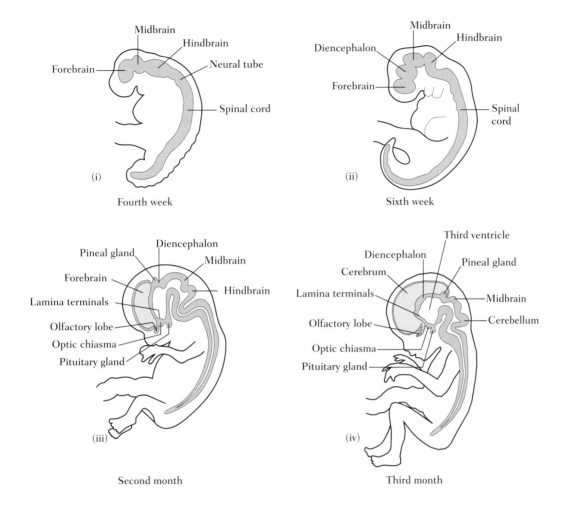

Figure 3.4: Embryological development of the central nervous system

The expanding and curling pattern of growth at the top of the neural tube is organized around the *lamina terminalis*. The lamina terminalis forms the front wall of the third ventricle (see Figure 3.2, page 41). This place acts as the natural fulcrum for the growth and development of the central nervous system. It remains as the place around which the craniosacral motion of the central nervous system is expressed throughout life, as long as there are no stressful influences which modify this motion.

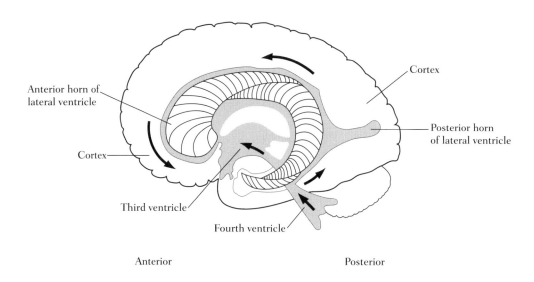

Anterior horn of
lateral ventricle

Cortex

Cortex

Posterior horn
of lateral ventricle

Third ventricle

Fourth ventricle

Anterior

Posterior

Figure 3.5: 'Ram's horn' motion of the brain

Inhalation and exhalation

The motility of the central nervous system is expressed as part of an integrated pattern of motion, associated with its surrounding membranes, bones and fluid. In health, all these tissues move in synchrony with each other.

As the central nervous system expresses the inhalation phase of the cranial rhythmic impulse, the brain rotates forwards towards the lamina terminalis, in a motion like the curling of a ram's horn (see Figure 3.5).[34] In inhalation, the front part of the cortex of the brain rotates anteriorly (towards the front) and inferiorly (footwards), and its back part rotates superiorly (towards the top of the head). At the same time, the brain widens from side to side, while shortening from front to back and from top to bottom. Simultaneously, the spinal cord rises while it widens from side to side and shortens from top to bottom. Dr Sutherland likened this motion of the central nervous system to a tadpole pulling up its tail.[35]

The opposite motion occurs during the exhalation phase, when there is an uncurling of the brain towards the back, a narrowing from side to side and a lengthening from front to back. The spinal cord lowers in exhalation, narrows, uncurls and elongates. In the inhalation phase, the ventricles of the brain widen from side to side and narrow from front to back (see Figure 3.6). This motion moves in synchrony with the welling up and rising of C.S.F. in the inhalation phase of its longitudinal fluctuation.

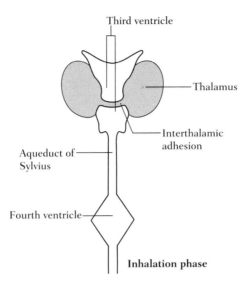

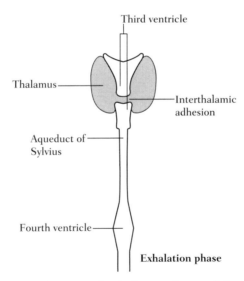

Figure 3.6: Inhalation and exhalation phases of the ventricles

God's drug store

The brain is one of the largest organs in the body. While it is widely recognized as the organ through which our thinking processes operate, this is now considered to be just a small part of its function. According to the psychologist Robert Ornstein and physician David Sobel, the main purpose of the brain is for the maintenance of health.[36] It has an extraordinary capacity to receive information, process it and act accordingly. It is the largest organ of secretion in the body, producing hundreds of chemicals according to our needs, including *neurotransmitters* used by individual nerve cells to communicate with each other. In this way, the brain maintains a balance between our internal physiology and our social worlds, environment, thoughts and feelings.

The brain makes countless adjustments, secretions and commands which it sends out to the rest of the body. Long before the chemicals of the brain had been scientifically analysed, Dr Still observed with great perception that, 'The brain is God's drug store having within all drugs, lubricating oils, opiates, acids, and every quality of drug that the wisdom of God thought necessary for human happiness and health.'[37] The motility expressed by the brain is thought to have an important influence on the way these chemicals are produced and distributed.

Maintenance of balance

In fact, the brain can be thought of as a collection of brains (see Figure 3.7). It is comprised of different parts, each with different functions, but all working together to maintain the balance of the body. Each part of the brain specializes in receiving or sending out particular messages and commands. However, if the different parts of the brain lose their ability to function in an integrated way, we may end up experiencing 'mixed messages'. The expression of primary respiratory motion is essential for maintaining the fluidity, integration and co-ordination of brain function.

Mind and body

Our psychological states have a critical influence on the physiology of the central nervous system. Some centres in the brain interpret thoughts and feelings, and translate these psychological states into physiological changes. These centres are collectively known as the *limbic system*, and are located near the centre of the brain. An emotion like fear, for example, can trigger the limbic system to initiate the release of certain chemicals, such as neuro-transmitters or hormones. These chemicals then produce a physiological response in the body.

If these psychological patterns are habitualized, the tissues of the central nervous system may become structurally organized accordingly. As a result, more permanent organic changes may take place. It is thought that particular psychological states can produce particular

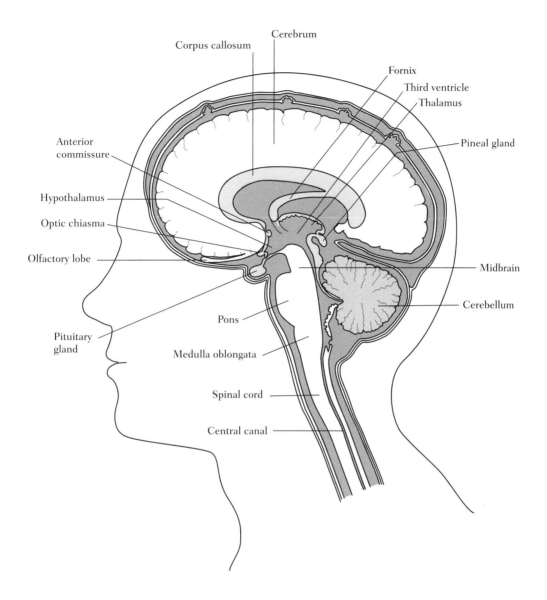

Figure 3.7: Mature brain: the basic parts

effects. For example, Stanley Keleman suggests that fear inhibits the brain, rage makes it over-active, sadness shrinks the brain, and defiance hardens it.[38] In this way, mental-emotional patterns directly translate into body patterning. As this principle holds true throughout the whole body, we will look at this subject in more depth a little later (see Chapter 8).

The ventricles

The ventricles are an inter-connecting system of cavities in the brain, filled with cerebrospinal fluid (C.S.F.). The ventricles are the remains of the hollow neural tube around which the nervous system developed in the embryo. C.S.F. is produced in the ventricles. The majority of C.S.F. is secreted by the choroid plexi located in the two large lateral ventricles contained in each hemisphere of the brain. However, some C.S.F. is also produced in the third and fourth ventricles, which are located below the lateral ventricles (see Figure 3.2, page 41). The ventricles act as storage areas for C.S.F. and its inherent healing potency.

Third ventricle

It is considered that C.S.F. is potentized with the Breath of Life mainly in the third ventricle.[39] It is here that the biodynamic forces of the Breath of Life become transmuted into the fluids. It's no coincidence that the walls of the third ventricle contain some of the most crucial nerve centres for the physiological balance of the body. The significance of this remarkable region has been recognized in many spiritual and traditional health care systems.

In the Indian and Tibetan systems of medicine, the third ventricle is traditionally considered to be the site of the primary energy centre of the body. This is known as the *ajana chakra* in Sanskrit. A chakra is a gateway through which energy passes. In these systems of healing, the ajana chakra is considered to distribute our most essential quality of energy. As Franklyn Sills points out, 'The Chinese call this centre the "true field of elixir" or the "true Niwan", or enlightened centre.'[40] Harish Johari, in his book on chakras, refers to the region around the third ventricle as the 'cave of Brahmin',[41] a place yogis go to during meditation.

The third ventricle is shaped like an inner tyre or a hollow flattened doughnut with a solid centre (formed by part of the thalamus of the brain). It is located at the centre of the brain, surrounded by the tissues of the hypothalamus, thalamus and basal ganglia. These are vitally important structures for processing information and regulating the body.

Pituitary and pineal glands

The walls of the third ventricle also contain both the pituitary and pineal glands. The pituitary gland is called the 'master gland' of the hormonal system, as it controls many other hormonal glands. It responds to messages received from the hypothalamus, located just above it, by releasing hormones which govern growth, sexual development, reproduction, blood sugar and stress responses. The rhythmic cycles of primary respiratory motion are thought to play an essential role in regulating the secretion of these pituitary hormones.

The obscurely functioning pineal gland is located at the back wall of the third ventricle. Much mystery still surrounds this gland, but it is known that it regulates the reproductive system and our biological clock. According to many spiritual traditions, the pineal gland is considered to be the seat of the soul. Interestingly, in adulthood crystals form in the pineal gland, sometimes referred to as 'brain sand'. Although no clear purpose for these crystals has been proven, they may function like many other types of crystal, i.e. as amplifiers of energy. They may assist in the uptake of potency of the Breath of Life, as it enters the C.S.F.

Dynamo motion

Much newly formed C.S.F. enters the third ventricle from the lateral ventricles, through openings in the front part of its roof. It then tends to circulate around the solid hub of the third ventricle, in a motion which has been likened to that of a dynamo (see Figure 3.8). It is thought that during this circulation, the potency of the Breath of Life is taken up in the C.S.F. Therefore, the third ventricle is considered as an important junction between the primary energy centre of the body and C.S.F. Freshly potentized C.S.F. immediately comes into contact with all the vital organs contained around the walls of the third ventricle.

Fourth ventricle

The fourth ventricle is located below the third ventricle, and connected to it by a long narrow channel called the *Aqueduct of Sylvius*. The fourth ventricle is a rhomboid-shaped cavity filled with cerebrospinal fluid (C.S.F.). It is also of great importance because its walls contain many of the major nerve centres of the body, including those which control lung breathing ('secondary respiration'), blood circulation, digestion, elimination, homeostasis and 10 of the 12 cranial nerves. These tissues, vital for physiological functioning, likewise become bathed with freshly formed and potentized C.S.F., carrying the ordering principle of the Breath of Life.

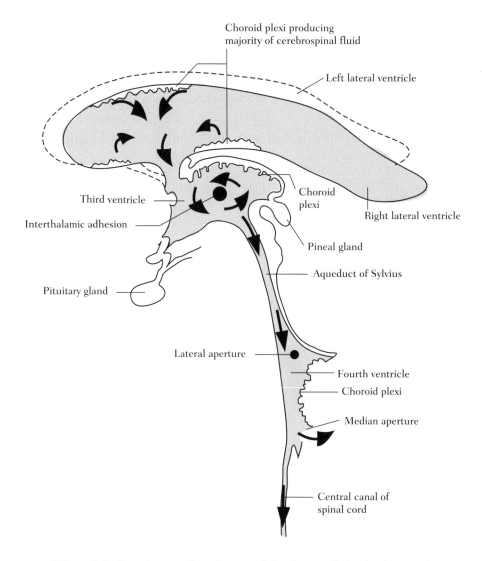

Figure 3.8: Circulation of cerebrospinal fluid around the third ventricle

3) The Mobility of the Reciprocal Tension

Membrane System

The central nervous system is contained within a system of connective tissues, called *meninges*. In all, there are three layers of meninges and they are an integral part of the primary respiratory mechanism (see Figure 3.9).

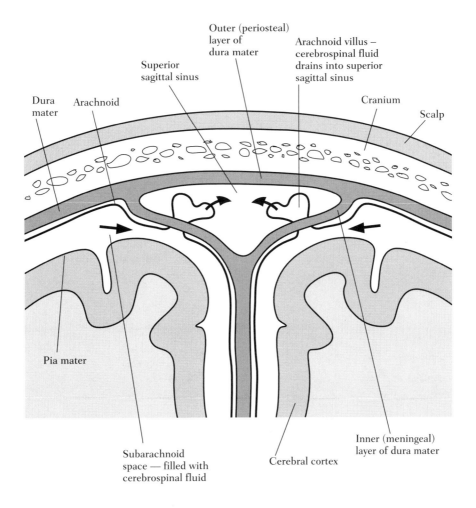

Figure 3.9: Cranial meninges and the formation of a venous sinus
(frontal section through the brain)

The inner layer of meninges closely follows all the contours and convolutions of the brain and spinal cord, like 'cling film' (plastic wrap). This layer is called the *pia mater* and is very thin and delicate.

The middle layer of meninges is called the *arachnoid* (because it resembles a spider's web) and is also thin and delicate. The arachnoid and pia mater are connected by thin strands of tissue, but there is a space between them called the subarachnoid space. It is within the sub-arachnoid space that C.S.F. circulates around the central nervous system.

The dural system

The outer layer of meninges is called the *dura mater*. *Dura* means 'strong' and *mater* means 'mother' ... so this tissue is considered a strong mother! This tough and fibrous membrane is, itself, formed of two layers which are largely fused together. However, at certain points in the skull the two layers of dura separate from each other. The inner *meningeal* layer splits away, while the outer *periosteal* layer adheres to the internal surfaces of cranial bones. At the places where the meningeal layer splits away, folds of tissue are created, forming partitions of the brain. These folds of dural membrane create strong vertical and horizontal sheets of tissue which help to regulate the motion of the primary respiratory mechanism. Furthermore, where the layers of dura separate, venous sinuses are formed (see Figure 3.9). These important channels drain both blood and reabsorbed cerebrospinal fluid from the head.

The continuous system of connective tissue formed from dural membranes is called the *reciprocal tension membrane system* (see Figure 3.10).

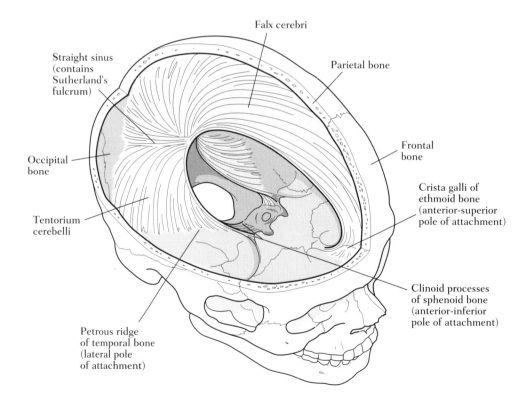

Figure 3.10: Cranial reciprocal tension membranes

Vertical partitions

There are two vertical partitions made of dura. The large upper vertical sheet of tissue, called the *falx cerebri*, separates the right and left cerebral hemispheres. It is a sickle-shaped membrane which traverses the underside of the skull from front to back. At the front, the falx cerebri is attached to the ethmoid bone (see Figure 3.10). It then passes beneath the frontal bone, runs under the suture between the two parietal bones and attaches at the back to the occipital bone. At the back it meets the horizontal partitions of dural membrane at an important junction in which the *straight sinus* is formed.

The *falx cerebelli* is a smaller vertical partition beneath the straight sinus, separating the right and left hemispheres of the cerebellum. It is attached by a dense ring of connective tissue to the *foramen magnum*, a large opening in the floor of the occipital bone through which the lower part of the brainstem and top of the spinal cord exit the skull. The ring of tissue around the foramen magnum is then continuous with a long tube of membrane which surrounds the spinal cord, the *spinal dura*.

Horizontal partitions

The horizontal folds of dural membrane separate the upper and lower portions of the brain, forming a partition between the cerebrum and the cerebellum. This tissue has two 'leaves' which form a tent-like structure across the back part of the skull. It is called the *tentorium cerebelli*. At its front end, the tentorium attaches to the sphenoid bone (see Figure 3.10). At the sides, it is attached to the inner ridges of the temporal bones and to a small part of the parietal bones. At the back, it attaches to the internal surface of the occipital bone. The two leaves of the horizontal tentorium meet with the vertical falx cerebri at the straight sinus in the midline.

Reciprocal tension motion

Dr Sutherland named these tissues the 'reciprocal tension membrane system' because they are maintained in a state of constant tension during all of their movements. As the dura is both continuous and relatively inelastic, any motion which takes place in one part of the system is easily transferred to another. In this way, the reciprocal tension membranes function as a unified system. Craniosacral motion is expressed through this system as a tensile pushing and pulling motion, first in one direction and then in another.

These membranes form an integral part of cranial rhythmic motion. During each phase of inhalation, the falx cerebri shifts anteriorly towards its attachment at the front and curls in on itself, narrowing from front to back (see Figure 3.11). The smaller falx cerebelli also narrows from front to back. Meanwhile, the tentorium flattens out and widens from side to side. It also moves forwards and rises where it attaches to the sphenoid bone at the front. The motion of these membranes coincides with a general narrowing from front to back and widening from side to side of the cranium during inhalation.

In the exhalation phase the opposite motion occurs. The falx cerebri uncurls, moves posteriorly and lengthens from front to back. Meanwhile, the tentorium narrows from side to side and becomes more 'domed', as it takes on more of a tent-shape again.

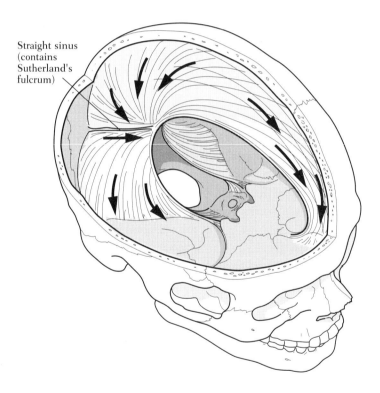

Straight sinus (contains Sutherland's fulcrum)

Figure 3.11: Inhalation/flexion phase of reciprocal tension membranes

Sutherland's fulcrum

The junction formed at the meeting place of the falx cerebri, the tentorium cerebelli and the falx cerebelli (i.e. the location of the straight sinus) contains *Sutherland's fulcrum* (see Figure 3.10, page 58). A fulcrum has been described as 'a point of rest on which a lever moves and from which it gets its power'.[42] Sutherland's fulcrum acts as the leverage point or pivot around which the reciprocal tension membranes express their craniosacral motion. The different partitions of the reciprocal tension membrane system can be thought of as suspending from this important fulcrum.

Sutherland's fulcrum is significant for the balanced motion of the reciprocal tension membrane system. It is a moving fulcrum which shifts up and down along the angle of the straight sinus during the cycles of craniosacral motion. It moves anteriorly and superiorly during inhalation, and posteriorly and inferiorly during exhalation. Any restrictions of motion which affect the balance of this dynamic, shifting fulcrum can upset the functioning of the entire reciprocal tension membrane system.

Integrated motion

In the early stages of our development, the reciprocal tension membranes are formed from the same embryonic tissue (mesenchym) as cranial bones. Part of this tissue hardens during the first few years of life to form cranial bones, and part of it remains as the dural membranes inside the skull. Therefore, the dural membranes and cranial bones can be seen as different elements within a continuity of tissue. In their expression of craniosacral motion, these bones and membranes act together as an integrated unit of function. Because these membranes are relatively inelastic, any pull or strain has a direct effect on the motion of cranial bones, and vice versa. Consequently, the reciprocal tension membranes have often been described as helping to transmit and guide the motion of cranial bones.

Recognizing the synchronized motion between cranial bones and membranes, Dr Sutherland referred to their restriction as a 'membranous-articular strain'.[43] It is not possible to have a strain in one without involving the other. As the brain is enclosed and partitioned by the dural membranes, its shape (and function) can be influenced by them. Membranous-articular strains can thus limit the motility of the central nervous system, the motion of cer-ebrospinal fluid, and the passage of fluid through the venous sinus system. The functioning of numerous cranial nerves which pass through the reciprocal tension membranes can also be affected. In fact, freedom of motion in the reciprocal tension membrane system is necessary for the proper functioning of all other aspects of the primary respiratory mechanism, which are either enclosed within it or directly attached to it.

The core link

The spinal dura is firmly attached to the occiput by the ring of connective tissue around the foramen magnum. From this point downwards it hangs quite freely, encircling the spinal cord, until it reaches the bottom of the spine. Here it is firmly attached to the second vertebral segment of the sacrum (S2) (see Figure 3.12). However, the 'dural tube' usually has some small slips of tissue which connect it to the second and third vertebrae of the neck, but these attachments do not fix it firmly to these points. The dural tube provides protection for the spinal cord and acts as a container for the inner layers of the meninges and the enclosed cerebrospinal fluid (C.S.F.).

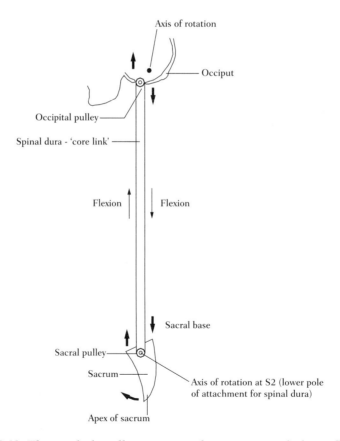

Figure 3.12: The core link; pulley-motion as the sacrum is rocked into flexion

As the spinal dura is relatively inelastic, it is a medium through which forces can be easily transmitted between the occiput at its top end and the sacrum below. The spinal dura thus provides an important link between the craniosacral motion of the pelvis and the cranium. This connection was called the *core link* by Dr Sutherland.[44]

During the inhalation phase of the cranial rhythmic impulse, the spinal dura rises, following the upward movement of Sutherland's fulcrum. The opposite happens in the exhalation phase. Dr John Upledger describes a pulley-like motion, during which the occiput and sacrum are reciprocally rocked into their craniosacral motion by the spinal dura.[45] When the occiput expresses its craniosacral motion in inhalation, the front part of the foramen magnum rises up. This exerts a pull up along the front side of the dural tube, raising the front side of the sacrum and rocking it into flexion (see Figure 3.12). In the exhalation phase, a pull is transmitted along the back side of the dural tube, rocking the sacrum into extension.

However, the dural tube can lose its natural ability to glide freely within the spinal canal. This can affect the motion of the sacrum, cranial bones and spinal vertebrae, the circulation of C.S.F, and can cause irritation of the spinal cord. This type of problem commonly results from a whiplash injury or other kinds of back strain.

Summary

Here's a summary of the natural motion of the different parts of the reciprocal tension membrane system. During the inhalation phase of the cranial rhythmic impulse:

- the falx cerebri shifts anteriorly towards its attachment at the ethmoid bone at the front, and shortens from front to back
- the falx cerebelli shortens from front to back
- the tentorium moves anteriorly, flattens and widens
- the membrane system as a whole moves up and shortens from top to bottom
- the spinal dural tube rises
- this motion has its pivot around Sutherland's fulcrum, located along the straight sinus. This is a moving, dynamic fulcrum which shifts position during the cycles of craniosacral motion.

During the exhalation phase, the opposite motion occurs.

An exercise

To illustrate the integrated motion of the dural membrane system, imagine that your whole body represents these membranes. Stand up with your knees slightly bent and your arms partly outstretched at the sides. Imagine that your legs and trunk are the spinal membranes, your head and neck is the falx cerebri, and your forehead is where the front of the falx cerebri attaches to the ethmoid bone. Your arms represent the tentorium. To demonstrate how the membrane system moves in its inhalation phase, slowly straighten your knees and, as your body rises, bend your head forwards and down so that your forehead curls slightly backwards, as you tuck in your chin. At the same time, spread your arms wider from side to side.

Then, to demonstrate the exhalation phase, bend your knees to represent the lowering of the spinal dura. Uncurl your head, thus mimicking the action of the falx cerebri, and bring your arms closer to your body, following the motion of the tentorium. Interestingly, these movements are similar to some ancient Chi Kung exercises, which apparently follow the natural designs of the body.[46]

4) The Motion of Cranial Bones

Dr Sutherland began his investigations into primary respiratory motion after recognizing the importance of cranial bony movement for our physiological functioning. There are 22 bones which make up the adult human skull. Eight of these form the cranium which encloses and protects the brain, the 'treasure in the citadel' (see Figure 3.13).[47] Fourteen bones form the face (see Figure 3.14). In addition, there are three tiny bones (ossicles) in each ear. The eight cranial bones are:

1	frontal bone
2–3	parietal bones (2)
4–5	temporal bones (2)
6	occipital bone
7	sphenoid bone
8	ethmoid bone.

The 14 facial bones are:

1–2	nasal bones (2)
3–4	maxillae (2)
5–6	zygomatic bones (2)

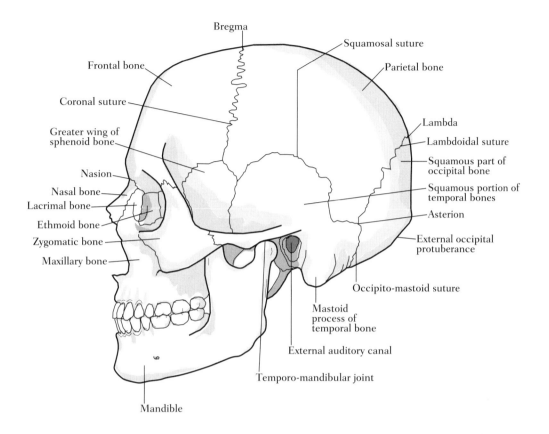

Figure 3.13: Bones of the skull – side view

7	mandible
8–9	lacrimal bones (2)
10–11	palatine bones (2)
12–13	inferior nasal conchae (2)
14	vomer.

In accordance with the Greek legend, the cranial bones are carried upon the shoulders of *atlas*, the name of the uppermost vertebra of the neck. The individual bones of the skull articulate with each other by a variety of differently shaped joints, which allow for various kinds of movement. These specialized articulations in the cranium are called *sutures*. It was while examining the design of these sutures that Dr Sutherland first had the insight that they were intended for motion. As Dr Magoun points out,

Why should there be articular surfaces at all if not for movement? Indeed the only factor physiologically capable of maintaining such joint surfaces throughout life ... is motion.[48]

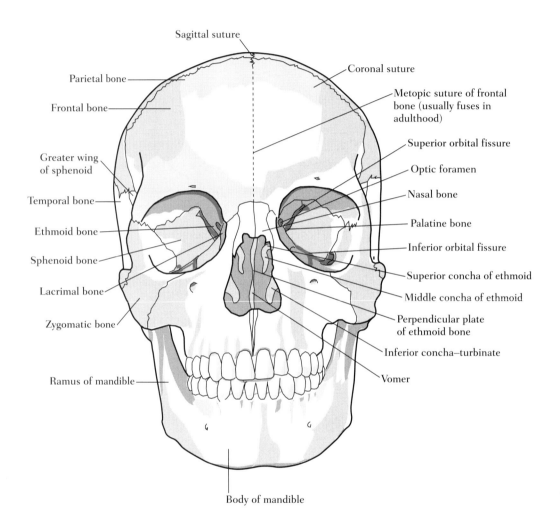

Figure 3.14: Bones of the face – anterior view

Formation of sutures

At the time of our birth, cranial bones still largely consist of either membrane or cartilage, and their sutures have not yet formed. Many sutures do not properly develop until about six years of age. The particular design that a suture acquires helps to determine the motion that can take place. However, there is also evidence to suggest that their design is at least partly formed as a consequence of the motion they express.[49] In other words, the bones form according to how they function. This reflects one of the key principles in osteopathic medicine – the structure and function of the body are reciprocally interrelated (see Chapter 4).

Some sutures are bevelled, with bones meeting each other at angled surfaces (see Figure 1.1, page 3). This design allows for a gliding or separating motion. Other sutures are serrated or corrugated, which allows for separation and a variety of hinge-like motions. Others are formed like sockets, allowing for rotatory or gliding motions. The shape of these 'articular gears'[50] is particular to each individual, and a unique expression of individual function. I have examined many skull specimens and have never seen two bones that are alike.

The bones of the adult skull fit together like an intricate jigsaw, producing over 100 sutural articulations. They are like the tectonic plates of the earth's crust, which shift on the earth's surface according to deeper forces which make them move.

Axes of rotation

The craniosacral motion of each bone is organized around an imaginary line, called an *axis of rotation*. All the bones of the body express their craniosacral motion in specific ways around a particular axis. An axis can be located in any of three planes (see Figure 3.15):

1   anterior-posterior axis (i.e. an imaginary line from front to back)
2   horizontal axis (i.e. an imaginary line from side to side)
3   vertical axis (i.e. an imaginary line from top to bottom).

To help picture each of these axes of rotation, take a pencil – this is going to play the part of the axis. First, hold the pencil so that the two ends point from your front to back. Then take a small piece of paper and fold a crease along the middle of the paper. Rest the crease of the folded paper on the pencil and rotate it over the pencil. This is how motion occurs around an anterior-posterior axis. If you then hold the pencil pointing from side to side (i.e. left to right), this provides a horizontal axis of rotation for the piece of paper. Finally, hold the pencil pointing from top to bottom to see how motion occurs around a vertical axis (don't

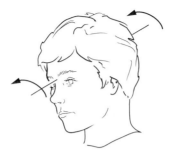

i) Side bending to the right
   around an anterior-posterior axis

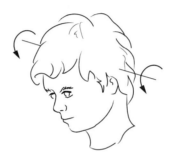

ii) Forward bending around
    a horizontal axis

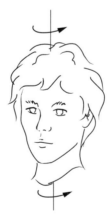

iii) Rotation to the left around
     a vertical axis

Figure 3.15: Axes of rotation

forget to keep hold of the paper for this one!). In practice, many bones move around a combination of these axes.

Midline bones

The terms 'flexion and extension' are used to describe the craniosacral motion of all the single, midline bones of the body. These motions occur around a horizontal axis of rotation. During the inhalation phase of craniosacral motion, all single midline bones move into flexion. During the exhalation phase, they move into extension.

To give an example, during inhalation the occiput rocks into flexion around a horizontal axis of rotation located just above the foramen magnum (see Figure 3.16). In this motion, the front part (basilar portion) of the occiput moves up, while the back part (squamous portion) moves down. During the exhalation phase, the occiput rocks back into extension: its front part moves down and its back part moves up.

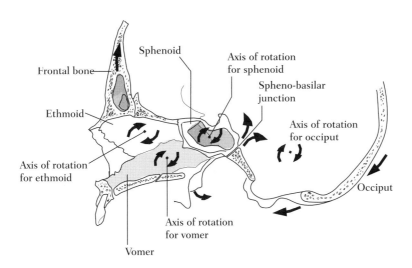

Figure 3.16: Flexion of midline cranial bones

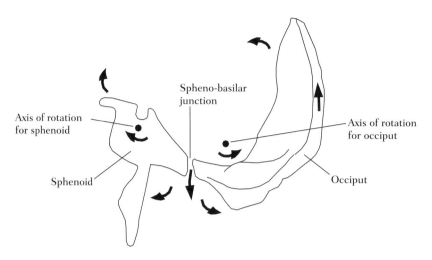

Figure 3.17: Extension of the sphenoid and occiput

Spheno-basilar junction

The sphenoid bone and occiput form most of the floor of the cranium. They meet at a carti-laginous joint called the *spheno-basilar junction*. This joint allows for minimal degrees of motion, even though it fuses in adulthood. Dr Sutherland designated the terms 'flexion and extension' to describe the motion which occurs at the underside of these two bones (see Figures 3.16 and 3.17). Flexion refers to a narrowing of the angle between the sphenoid and occiput at their underside, and extension refers to an increasing of this angle.

As the sphenoid and occiput express their flexion phase of craniosacral motion, both the greater wings of the sphenoid and the back part of the occiput move down, towards the feet (see Figure 3.16). At the same time, the spheno-basilar junction rises. During the extension phase, the greater wings of the sphenoid and the back part of the occiput rise, while the spheno-basilar junction lowers (see Figure 3.17).

The spheno-basilar junction is considered to be the natural fulcrum or pivot of all other cra-nial bony movements. In fact, the sphenoid is considered to be the cog from which all other bones 'gear off'. The craniosacral motion of all the other midline bones in the body is named as flexion and extension in relationship to the motion at the spheno-basilar junction.

The other midline bones of the body follow the motion of the occiput, and express their flex-ion and extension by rotating in the *opposite* direction to the sphenoid (see Figure 3.16). In the skull, the other midline bones are the frontal, ethmoid, vomer and mandible. They all move into flexion and extension around their individual horizontal axes of rotation.

Importance of the sphenoid

The sphenoid is endowed with considerable importance in the craniosacral concept. It forms a large part of the anterior floor of the cranium, as well as the back portion of the eye sockets. Many cranial nerves pass through or alongside the sphenoid, and so their function can be influenced by it. Problems with eyesight and facial pain commonly result from the irritation of these nerves. The balanced expression of primary respiratory motion in this area is necessary for the healthy function of these nerves.

The pituitary gland sits in a dip in the sphenoid bone, called the *sella turcica* or 'Turkish saddle'. The pituitary is gently rocked in its saddle during the phases of craniosacral motion. This rocking motion is considered to encourage the balanced release of pituitary hormones, by helping to 'milk' the gland.[51] I have worked with many patients with various types of hormonal disorders, such as infertility, chronic stress and menstrual problems. Many of these people have responded well to craniosacral work at the sphenoid bone, which has helped to balance their pituitary function.

Furthermore, the sphenoid has a deep connection to the functioning of consciousness. Hugh Milne suggests that it is the seat of our 'inner eye', concerned with the ability to maintain spiritual vision in our lives.[52] If the sphenoid becomes restricted in its capacity to express craniosacral motion, it may restrict the ability of our consciousness to expand. This condition is often found in states of depression. When motion of the sphenoid is open and free, it can allow for a depth and spaciousness of inner vision.

Paired bones

The terms 'external rotation' and 'internal rotation' describe the craniosacral motion of all the paired bones in the body. In the cranium, these movements mainly occur around an anterior-posterior axis (front to back). During the inhalation phase of craniosacral motion, all paired bones move into external rotation. During the exhalation phase, they move into internal rotation.

The paired bones of the cranium are the temporals, parietals, frontal, maxillae, palatines, zygomae, lacrimals, nasal bones and nasal conchae. The frontal bone is included in this list because, as well as being a midline bone, it also functions in the same way as paired bones. This is because it originates as two bones, which are divided by a suture along the midline, called the *metopic suture* (see Figure 3.14, page 66). The frontal bone usually fuses at this suture by about the age of six, although it remains unfused throughout life in about 10 per cent of the population. However, even when fused, the remnant of this suture allows for some internal and external rotation. Further descriptions of the craniosacral motion of each bone can be found in any one of the specialized textbooks on the subject.[53]

Cranial motility

In addition to the mobility which takes place at their sutures, cranial bones also express a motility. Motility is the direct result of primary respiratory motion being expressed from within; the Breath of Life creating an inner 'breathing'. During the inhalation phase, bones express this motility by expanding and widening from side to side. In exhalation, there is a narrowing from side to side. Motility is a fundamental prerequisite to the healthy functioning of a bone. As Dr James Jealous observes, 'Before a bone can have a relationship with another bone on either side of it, it must first have a relationship within itself.'[54] The balanced expression of both mobility and motility is evidence of that bone's healthy functioning.

Inter-connections

All the bones of the skull express a specific pattern of craniosacral motion, but function in relationship to each other, like inter-connected wheel cogs. These bones can be visualized as floating 'like corks on the tide', driven in their motion by a deeper tide and regulated by their underlying membranes. As the dural membranes express their craniosacral motion, they help to pull the cranial bones into a rhythmic motion. Bone and membrane thus move together with synchronicity. Consequently, cranial bones can be thought of as more solid places in this continuity of tissue. They are frequently used by craniosacral practitioners as 'handles' for the palpation and treatment of any problems which involve the underlying reciprocal tension membranes.

If all these tissues are able to express their mobility and motility freely, they allow for the permeation of the Breath of Life and its ordering principle. However, as a result of their connection to other tissues, restrictions of cranial bones can influence the functioning of numerous physiological processes elsewhere. Particularly, the fluctuation of cerebrospinal fluid and motility of the central nervous system may be affected. Similarly, inertia which starts in other regions may lead to a restriction of cranial bones.

All bones carry a significance linked to their individual location and function. For example, the maxillary bones at the front of the face are closely connected to the functioning of the eyes, nose, sinuses and mouth. However, stressful forces that impede a bone's primary respiratory motion may disturb its ability to function healthily. While each bone has importance, the temporal bones are discussed in more detail below, to give an example of what can happen.

Temporal bones

The two temporal bones are located at the sides of the head and also form part of the cranial floor (see Figure 3.13, page 65). They have an exquisite and intricate design. It was the bevelled sutures of the temporals which first struck Dr Sutherland as being like the gills of a fish, intended for primary respiratory motion.[55] The temporals articulate with seven other cranial bones:

1	the occiput
2	the sphenoid
3–4	the two parietal bones
5–6	the two zygomae and
7	the mandible.

The temporal bones fill the wedge-shaped spaces between the occiput and sphenoid, and sometimes become jammed together with these other two bones. Many important structures may get compressed as a result. Physical trauma, such as a long or difficult birth, is one common cause of this.

Once fluid has drained through the venous sinus system, about 95 per cent of it exits from the head via two small holes, called *jugular foramina*. These are located in the sutures formed between the temporal bones and the occiput. If either of the jugular foramina becomes narrowed, fluid drainage from the head can get impaired. Congestive headaches and tiredness commonly result. Furthermore, the jugular foramina contain three pairs of cranial nerves, including the widely influential vagus nerves. The function of these nerves can also be irritated by compression (see also Chapter 5, Cranial Nerves). Craniosacral treatment to help disengage these sutures can bring about the effective relief of cranial congestion or nerve irritation.

Furthermore, the temporal bones contain the organs of hearing and balance. These faculties can become disturbed when primary respiratory motion is compromised. Problems such as hearing difficulties, tinnitus and dizziness may result. The *auditory tubes*, which stabilize air pressure in the ears, can also become affected. This often creates a tendency to ear infections.

The temporal bones also function in close continuity with the reciprocal tension membrane system. The tentorium cerebelli attaches along the *petrous ridges* at the inside of the temporal bones, and important venous sinuses are contained within these membranes (see Figure 3.9, page 57). Venous sinus drainage, as well as problems referred through the reciprocal tension membranes, may result from patterns of inertia.

The mandible (jaw bone) articulates with the temporal bones at joints located just in front of the ears (see Figure 3.13, page 65). These are the most used joints in the body, brought into action every time we eat, drink, talk or yawn. The position and mobility of the temporal bones directly influences the functioning of the *temporo-mandibular* joints. A wide range of clinical symptoms can result from problems which affect these joints, including jaw pain, clicking of the jaw, restricted opening of the mouth, dental problems, headaches, neck and shoulder pain, hearing problems, difficulty swallowing, tinnitus, dizziness and facial pain.

In recognition of the widespread consequences that difficulties with the temporal bones may create, Dr Sutherland referred to them as 'mischief makers'.[56] However, this is a two-way relationship, because these bones not only influence, but can also be influenced by, other parts of the primary respiratory mechanism.

5) The Involuntary Motion of the Sacrum

Between the Iliac Bones of the Pelvis

The sacrum is a large, triangular-shaped bone made up of five fused vertebrae. It fits between the two iliac bones of the pelvis, forming the base upon which the spinal column rests. It articulates with the bones of the pelvis via *sacro-iliac joints* on each side. The sacral (i.e. 'sacred') bone is thus the foundation of the spine and supports the weight of the whole trunk. As such, it plays an important role in the healthy workings of the rest of the spine. Any inertia which affects the sacrum can alter the functioning of vertebrae higher up. This is a common cause of backache.

The sacrum is firmly strapped to the pelvic bones and to the vertebrae just above by strong bands of connective tissue, called *ligaments*. Nevertheless, the sacro-iliac joints are sufficiently flexible to allow for small degrees of motion. A *voluntary* motion occurs during the actions of walking, running, etc., and an *involuntary* motion occurs during the different phases of primary respiratory motion. There are no muscles which connect the sacrum to the pelvis, so any motion (voluntary or involuntary) which takes place here has to be created by other causes.

As above, so below

As we noted, the dural tube is firmly attached at its upper end to the occiput, but then has no firm attachments until it reaches the second segment of the sacrum. This 'core-link' makes the sacrum an integral part of the primary respiratory mechanism. The relatively inelastic dural tube helps to transmit craniosacral motion between the occiput and the sacrum (see Figure 3.12, page 62). As the occiput rocks into flexion and extension, so the sacrum moves in synchrony. In addition, this involuntary motion of the sacrum is gently impelled by the longitudinal fluctuation of cerebrospinal fluid. Because the sacrum is directly connected to the rest of the primary respiratory mechanism, its motion may easily influence or become affected by these other regions.

Sacral motion

As the sacrum is a single midline bone, its flexion and extension are expressed around a horizontal axis. The axis of rotation for this movement is located at the second sacral segment (S2), where the dural tube is attached. Also, as a single midline bone the sacrum rotates in the opposite direction to the sphenoid. When it moves into flexion, the upper part of the sacrum (called the *sacral base*) rotates posteriorly and superiorly, while its lower part moves anteriorly (towards the pubic symphysis) and inferiorly (see Figure 3.12). Motility is expressed at the sacrum as a widening and uncurling of the bone in the inhalation phase. In exhalation, it narrows and curls up.

Nerve irritation

Nerves which regulate the organs of reproduction and elimination emerge through small openings in the sacrum. These nerves can become irritated if they get compressed, which could happen if the sacrum becomes locked in a certain position. Irritation of the sacral nerves may produce gynaecological, reproductive, bowel or urinary tract disorders. Nerves also emerge from the sacrum to form the great sciatic nerve, which controls many muscles of the leg. If this nerve becomes irritated, it can produce the painful symptoms of *sciatica*.

The sacrum can be subject to a wide range of influences, psychological as well as physical, which can disturb its motion. Because of the sacrum's location and function, feelings of insecurity, issues of 'grounding', experiences such as sexual abuse or a lack of support are often reflected in its pattern of craniosacral motion.

THE WHOLE BODY

All parts in the whole body obey the one eternal law of life and motion.[57]
DR A. T. STILL

The five core aspects of the primary respiratory mechanism are in direct relationship to the dural membrane system, and are all located along the midline of the body. However, the expression of primary respiratory motion is not limited to these core tissues.

Connective tissues

One of the basic principles of craniosacral work is that everything in the body is connected to everything else. The connective tissues of the body are important parts of this integrated system. There is a continuous network of connective tissue from head to toe, and from the core of the primary respiratory mechanism to the periphery of the body. These tissues express craniosacral motion in certain specific ways.

The dural membrane system is a part of the body's unbroken chain of connective tissue. These membranes are continuous with the lining (periosteum) inside the cranial bones and sacrum. Other connective tissues are continuous with the periosteum outside these bones. From attachments on the underside of the cranium, bands of connective tissue hang down, forming longitudinal compartments which traverse the length of the body. These longitudinal tissues hang from the cranial bones like great tubes which wrap the various organs and internal structures of the body (see Figure 3.18). Furthermore, as each nerve exits from the spinal canal it is enveloped in a 'sleeve' of tissue which is continuous with the dural tube of the spine (see Figure 3.19). Once these dural sleeves leave the spinal canal, they join up with the connective tissue network of the rest of the body, linking the core tissues of the primary respiratory mechanism with the body as a whole.

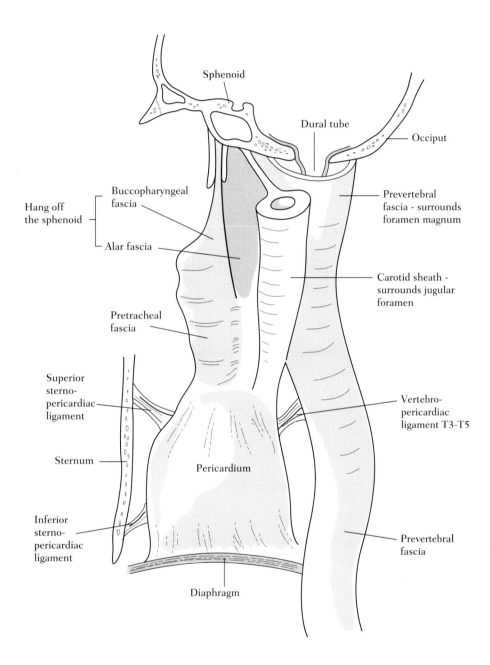

Figure 3.18: Connective tissues (fascia) hanging from the cranial floor[58]

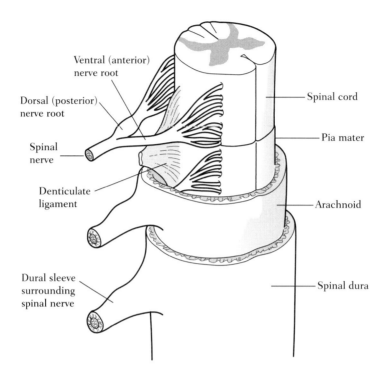

Ventral (anterior)
nerve root

Dorsal (posterior)
nerve root

Spinal
nerve

Denticulate
ligament

Dural sleeve
surrounding
spinal nerve

Spinal cord

Pia mater

Arachnoid

Spinal dura

Figure 3.19: Formation of spinal nerves with connective tissue coverings

Role of fascia

Fascia is a type of connective tissue found throughout the body. It is an organ of support which also helps to compartmentalize the different body structures. There is a superficial layer of fascia which immediately underlies the skin, and deeper layers which surround all the internal structures of the body. Each nerve, muscle, bone, vessel, gland and organ of the body is surrounded by deep fascia – as is each individual nerve fibre, muscle fibre and each group of fibres. In fact, every 'everything' in the body is surrounded by fascia. If you took away all the internal substance of the body, you would be left with a cast of each body part made of fascia.

The fascia around a muscle, nerve, organ, etc., determines the space that these structures take up, and so maintains their shape. In addition, fascia forms an integrating tissue system which unifies the body, connecting all parts together. It helps all areas of the body to work together in co-ordinated patterns of movement. Therefore, the structure and the function of each individual part, and of the body as a whole, is to some extent controlled by fascia. As a result, fascia has an important role in maintaining our health.

Fascial glide

In health, all the fascial compartments throughout the body glide in relationship to each other. The fluid found between the different fascial sheets helps to reduce any friction so that this gliding motion can more easily occur. This *fascial glide* occurs during our more pronounced voluntary movements and during our subtle primary respiratory motion. Fascial glide allows for each part of the body to move easily against its neighbour, and accommodates for the inner breathing or motility of each part. When there is no resistance provided by their surrounding fascia, all tissues have room to 'breathe' and are thus able to express their original matrix of health.

Fluidic nature

Fluid is everywhere in the body, with water making up an average of 65 per cent of total body weight. Our bodies are basically fluidic in nature.[59] Earlier, we noted that the potency of the Breath of Life is conducted through the body within its fluid medium. As potency is taken up in the fluid, it produces a rhythmic longitudinal fluctuation. This tide-like phenomenon is expressed by all fluids of the body, not only by cerebrospinal fluid (C.S.F.). While C.S.F. is considered to be the primary medium which carries the potency of the Breath of Life, this function is also shared by other fluids.

Connective tissues, too, are largely comprised of fluid. Connective tissue is formed of hollow *collagen* and *elastin* fibres which are meshed together in sheets. These fibres are contained within a *ground substance*, made up of fluid. The fluid ground substance can vary in density from being quite watery to having a thicker, more gel-like state. A variety of different tissue types are formed, dependent on the fluidic nature of the ground substance, and the quantity and arrangement of collagen and elastin fibres.

Interestingly, the ground substance in connective tissues has a very similar composition to C.S.F.[60] Furthermore, like C.S.F., the fluid within connective tissues also expresses a tide-like rhythmic motion. Claire Dolby D.O. remarks, 'In the cranial concept, at a core level cerebrospinal fluid expresses the potency of the Breath of Life within the dural membranes. In the whole body, interstitial and lymphatic fluids at a cellular level and a tissue level carry out this role.'[61]

Conductor of potency

Small amounts of C.S.F. gain exit from the spinal canal via the dural sleeves which surround the spinal nerves (see earlier section on C.S.F., pages 40–2). The hollow collagen fibres of these connective tissues have been shown to be the agency by which this occurs, helping to transport C.S.F. into the rest of the body.[62] This supports an original hypothesis by Dr Sutherland, that cerebrospinal fluid potentizes the whole body.

Through its internal network of collagen fibres, the fascia can be seen as one of the mechanisms by which the potency of the Breath of Life is conducted throughout the body. The founder of osteopathy, Dr Still, affirmed the importance of fascia when he wrote:

> *This philosophy has chosen the fascia as a foundation on which*
> *we stand ... By its action we live and by its failure we die ... The soul*
> *of man with all the streams of pure living water seems to dwell in*
> *the fascia of his body.*[63]

The ability of fascia to act as a carrier of potency is further suggested by research carried out by Dr Zvi Karni, a professor of Biological Engineering in Israel. He suggests that fascia is able to conduct electricity, so helping to transmit energy throughout the body.[64] Other researchers such as Herbert Frohlich[65] and Fritz Popp have demonstrated that a living cell, in fact, emits light across a wide variety of wavelengths and that this is an important way in which cells communicate with each other. According to Dr Will Wilson, 'In cancer the output of light is much reduced, thereby reducing the potential for cell to cell communication. Cancer cells act as if out of touch with the rest of the organism, proliferating uncontrollably. So, for cellular health it seems likely that a light-based communication system is needed.'[66] It is likely that contraction of fascial tissues interferes with their capacity to conduct electricity,[67] and perhaps also with their ability to transmit light at a cellular level. This may be an important cause of a fragmentation of function between different parts of the body.

Core and periphery

Fascia has the properties of being pliable, tough and yet also relatively inelastic. The effects of a pull or twist in one area can easily be transmitted to another. An imbalance or restriction of fascial glide in any part of the network can affect other regions, thereby reducing the ability of the body to express its craniosacral motion. Scars are one common cause of this.

Since the fascial sheaths of the body are continuous with the reciprocal tension membrane system, patterns of stress affecting fascia in the periphery of the body can feed back into the core of the primary respiratory mechanism, and vice versa. Inertia within the fascial network can also place pressure on the internal organs of the body. This can reduce their ability to express their inherent motility and health.

The body functions as an integrated system, with all parts moving and working in relationship to each other. Because of this, it's possible for a practitioner to put his hand on, say, a patient's foot and palpate how primary respiratory motion is being expressed through the whole body. When doing this it may even be possible to notice how tissues at the opposite end of the body are functioning. These principles will be explored further in the later chapter on diagnosis.

Longitudinal arrangement

The majority of fascia is organized in longitudinal bands along the length of the body.[68] If the Breath of Life is expressed in health and balance, these bands of connective tissue freely glide in relationship to each other and allow for the healthy transmission of craniosacral motion throughout the body.

Because of the predominantly longitudinal organization of fascia, craniosacral motion is largely transmitted longitudinally through the fascial network. This physical arrangement corresponds to the way energy moves through the body. In Chinese medicine, energy or *chi* is considered to largely traverse the body along longitudinal channels, called meridians.

Transverse diaphragms

However, there are four key areas of the body where significant transverse (horizontal) arrangements of tissue are located (see Figure 3.20). These *transverse diaphragms* are:

1 the cranial base
2 the thoracic inlet
3 the respiratory diaphragm
4 the pelvic floor.

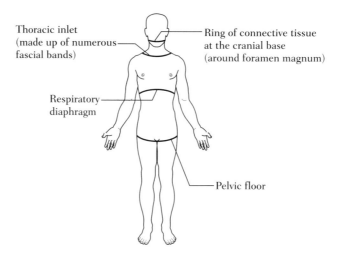

Figure 3.20: Major transverse diaphragms

The areas where transverse fascia is found in the body are essentially places of transition. They help to compartmentalize the different body cavities. For example, the respiratory diaphragm separates the abdomen from the chest, and the pelvic diaphragm creates the boundary of the pelvic floor.

When expressing their natural, unrestricted craniosacral motion, fluid and potency are free to move through the transverse diaphragms in a way which is similar to how water may spread along the contours of a funnel. However, contractions at the transverse diaphragms commonly act as sites of restriction to fascial glide and the expression of craniosacral motion. These transitionary areas have been noted by many 'body psychotherapists' as places where the flow of feelings and sensations often become blocked.[69] These places are where we may 'cut off' under stress, creating a fragmentation of function, say, between the legs and the trunk, the belly and the chest, or the head and the body.

Internal organs

The vitalizing forces of the Breath of Life are expressed in all bones, tissues, organs and vessels of the body. The internal organs of the body express their primary respiratory motion as a widening during inhalation and narrowing during exhalation. At the same time, the single organs (i.e. heart, stomach, bladder) express flexion and extension, while the paired organs (i.e. lungs, kidneys) move into external and internal rotation.

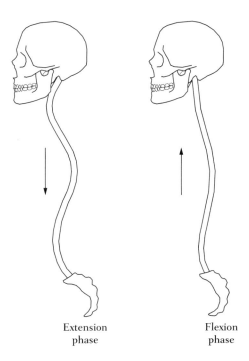

Extension
phase

Flexion
phase

Figure 3.21: Spinal curves in flexion and extension

Spinal mobility

The spine is the central column of support for the body. The spine's tone and flexibility are key elements in maintaining the balance of many functions in the body (see Figure 5.5, page 119). The spinal column expresses the micro-movements of craniosacral motion in addition to more apparent voluntary motions. As a whole, the spinal column tends to rise, while its curves uncurl in the inhalation/flexion phase. It then sinks and its curves become more pronounced in the extension phase (see Figure 3.21). Individual vertebrae express their craniosacral motion by subtly rocking into flexion and extension.

Many restrictions which affect the flexibility of the spine have at their root a condition of inertia involving primary respiratory motion. When primary respiratory motion is restored, the larger movements of the spine also tend to become freer. As an osteopath I see many patients with back problems. In the majority of these cases I find the craniosacral approach the most effective way of helping to restore mobility. It is also very gentle. It's now quite rare that I need to use other more physically invasive approaches, such as spinal manipulation or deep tissue massage.

Muscular motion

Muscles also express primary respiratory motion. Although not directly connected to the core of the primary respiratory mechanism, muscles that are attached to cranial bones or the sacrum can have an important influence. Contracted muscles may exert pressure on the core tissues of the body from the outside. Inertia affecting the muscular system sometimes needs to be addressed as a prerequisite to finding balance within the tissues of the primary respiratory mechanism.

Whole body craniosacral motion

The body as a whole expresses craniosacral motion as a widening from side to side in inhalation, followed by a narrowing in exhalation (see Figure 3.22). The limbs move into external and internal rotation and the feet move into dorsi-flexion and plantar flexion. Dorsi-flexion refers to a flexing motion at the ankle, during which the upper surface of the foot moves closer to the shin bone. Plantar flexion refers to a flexing motion in the other direction, when the upper surface of the foot moves further away from the shin bone, as when standing on tip-toe.

Summary of the Primary Respiratory System

The primary respiratory system refers to the whole range of subtle rhythms produced by the Breath of Life, as well as the ground of stillness from which this motion emerges. All aspects of primary respiratory motion (the long tide, mid-tide and cranial rhythmic impulse) help to convey the ordering principle of the Breath of Life. The cranial rhythmic impulse is expressed throughout the body as particular tissue movements called craniosacral motion. Other, slower tidal rhythms underlie this motion and are the essential forces behind it.

Primary respiratory motion carries our original matrix of health, an original intention for order and balance first seen during our embryological development. Therefore, there is a direct relationship between motion and health; all healthy tissues fully breathe with the Breath of Life, which maintains their order and integrity.

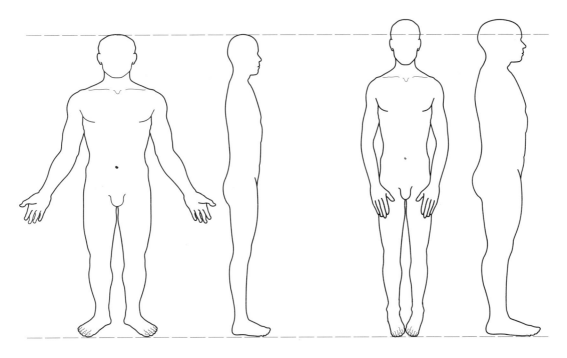

FLEXION/EXTERNAL ROTATION

- Body widens side to side
- Narrows front to back
- Shortens top to bottom
- Limbs externally rotate

EXTENSION/INTERNAL ROTATION

- Body narrows side to side
- Widens front to back
- Lengthens top to bottom
- Limbs internally rotate

Figure 3.22: Whole body craniosacral motion[70]

Summary of the Primary Respiratory Mechanism

The primary respiratory mechanism describes the tissues and fluids at the core of the body which play a key role in expressing the Breath of Life. The primary respiratory mechanism can be thought of as a car, with each part carrying out a different, yet vital function. The bones of the body move into flexion and extension and external and internal rotation like the cogs of the wheels. The reciprocal tension membranes are like the wheel axles, guiding the bones in their motion. The inhalation and exhalation of the central nervous system is like the piston of the engine; cerebrospinal fluid is the fuel. The potency of Breath of Life is the spark which ignites the fuel and moves the whole thing. The original matrix is the design. The driver is consciousness … and the shape of the bodywork gets conditioned by any traumatic influences![71]

Below is a summary of the particular ways the tissues of the body express their craniosacral motion.

Craniosacral Motion

Inhalation and exhalation are the specific terms used to describe the craniosacral motion of cerebrospinal fluid and the central nervous system.

Flexion/extension and external/internal rotation describe the craniosacral motion of bones, organs and membranes of the body (see Figure 3.23). All these motions are organized in relationship to the midline of our embryological development.

	Inhalation/flexion/ external rotation phase	Exhalation/extension/ internal rotation phase
Cerebrospinal fluid	Ascends longitudinally and spreads from side to side	Descends longitudinally and recedes from side to side
Central nervous system	Widens from side to side and shortens towards the front wall of the third ventricle	Narrows from side to side and lowers
Ventricles	Widen	Narrow
Falx cerebri and falx cerebelli	Narrows from front to back. Tentorium widens from side to side. Spinal dura rises	Lengthen from front to back. Tentorium narrows from side to side. Spinal dura lowers
Single midline bones	Move into flexion around a horizontal axis. Other bones rotate in opposite direction to the sphenoid	Move into extension around a horizontal axis. Other bones rotate in opposite direction to the sphenoid
Paired bones	Move into external rotation around specific anterior-posterior axes	Move into internal rotation around specific anterior-posterior axes (motion opposite to their external rotation)
Single organs	Move into flexion	Move into extension
Paired organs	Move into external rotation	Move into internal rotation
Feet	Externally rotate and dorsi-flex	Internally rotate and plantar-flex
Arms	Externally rotate	Internally rotate
Whole body	Widens from side to side and narrows from front to back	Narrows from side to side and widens from front to back

Figure 3.23: Craniosacral motion

4

THE INTELLIGENT
BODY

What is the body? That shadow of a shadow of your love, that somehow contains the whole universe.[1]

JELALUDDIN RUMI

KEY PRINCIPLES

All must have, and cannot act without the
highest known order of force, which submits to
the voluntary and involuntary commands of
life and mind, by which worlds are driven
and beings move.[2]
DR A. T. STILL

One of the principles of craniosacral practice is that nature is supremely intelligent and does not make mistakes. Nature always seeks balance, whatever the circumstances. This is not an idea born out of some act of faith, but something that can be seen operating throughout creation. The way the world turns, a forest regenerates or a wound heals are examples of this. Furthermore, it seems that nothing happens by accident – our health and happiness, as well as our disease and suffering, arise due to a certain set of causes and conditions. If we stop to consider, we may recognize how this intelligence gets played out in our own lives.

Science and art

The craniosacral approach is a way of facilitating health that has been developed by observing natural laws at work.[3] It is both a science and an art. As a science it involves 'the systematic observation of natural phenomena for the purpose of discovering laws governing these phenomena' (*Dorland's Medical Dictionary*).[4] As an art it involves the skilful application of these laws. Some of the key principles upon which this work is based will now be highlighted.

Many of the principles behind craniosacral work were originally outlined by Dr Andrew Taylor Still, a frontier doctor in 19th-century America. Dr Still developed the science of osteopathy after experiencing years of dissatisfaction with the inadequate and detrimental effects of the drug-based medicine which he initially practised.

Dr Still pointed out that, rather than addressing only materialistic phenomena, this approach works with nature's laws of 'matter, motion and mind'.[5] *Matter* refers to the body, the remarkable instrument into which life is expressed. Life is expressed as *motion*. *Mind* refers to the universal intelligence which flows through us.[6] Although encompassing subtle and often intangible realms of functioning, these phenomena are governed by natural laws which are as precise as any mechanistic law.[7]

Foundations of practice

Dr Still was perhaps the first to recognize the significant relationship between motion and health. As a young boy he used to suffer from headaches. One day while in his back garden he let his head lean back onto a suspended rope hammock. As he rested in this position, the swinging rope took the weight of his head, producing a gentle traction in his neck. He discovered that this measure soon relieved his headache and the nausea which accompanied it. As he described in his autobiography,

> *After that discovery I roped my neck whenever I felt one of those spells coming on. I followed that treatment for twenty years before the wedge of reason reached my brain, and I could see that I had suspended the action of the great occipital nerves, and given harmony to the flow of the arterial blood to and through the veins, and ease was the effect.*[8]

Dr Still recognized the importance of encouraging a free circulation of fluids within the body. He saw that this was a prerequisite to furnishing cells with their nutrients for health and removing toxins. Dr Still also realized that the motion of fluid enabled a free flow of 'life currents' through the body. He concluded that, 'Sickness is an effect caused by the stoppage of some supply of fluid or quality of life.'[9] He outlined three basic principles upon which the new science of osteopathy would be based:

1   Structure and function are reciprocally interrelated.
2   The body functions as a unit in health and disease.
3   The body is a self-healing mechanism.

THE RELATIONSHIP BETWEEN STRUCTURE AND FUNCTION

> *All living matter is subject to the 'LAW OF CHANGE' ... The relationship between structure and function is never constant. Both develop co-ordinately, one dependent upon the other, and this same interdependence holds true throughout every manifestation of life.*[10]
> CARTER H. DOWNING D.O.

Dr Still found that there is a close correspondence between the body's structural organization (i.e. anatomy) and the way in which we function (i.e. physiology). He noticed that restrictions of motion in the structural framework of the body affect its ability to receive the essential health-giving ingredients carried in the fluids.

The body's structure provides the container which determines what is able to flow through, in the same way that the flow of a river is determined by the course of its banks and whether there are any obstructions.

Reciprocal relationship

Furthermore, Dr Still realized that the relationship between structure and function is reciprocal – that is, each influences the other. Just as the body's structure governs its function, so also its function governs its structure. For example, if we regularly engage in a particular activity such as carrying a bag on one side or crossing one leg over the other, or if we have a poor work posture, the tissues of the body start to organize around these activities. Certain muscles may be used, while others are not. A particular structural pattern will be created, which then influences how we function. In this way, structure and function are mutually perpetuating, creating fixed patterns which become habitualized. As osteopath Charles Bowles summarizes, 'Function is structure in action; structure is function after action.'[11]

Primary respiratory function

Dr Sutherland's great contribution in this field was to recognize that the deepest relationship between structure and function is found in the primary respiratory system. At a core level, the functioning of the Breath of Life determines how our tissues become organized, like the contours of a river are determined by the flow of water which runs through it. However, again this is a reciprocal relationship – for the way the Breath of Life is able to manifest is also dependent upon our structural patterns.

Particular shapes and patterns in the body are created by the experiences we have in life. For instance, if faced with a stress or trauma, tissues tend to contract as part of a natural protective response. If these contractions remain unresolved, it results in prolonged states of inertia which restrict the vitalizing properties of the Breath of Life. This impedes the manifestation of our basic ordering principle in the tissues.

Effects of inertia

Inertial tissues influence many aspects of physiological functioning. To illustrate, let's say that a muscle goes into a contraction and remains in tension. This can cause joint stiffness, and also creates tension in the surrounding connective tissues. This restriction may start to impinge on blood vessels, reducing the circulation of arterial blood carrying oxygen and nutrients into the region. It may also interfere with the removal of waste products and toxins via the venous and lymphatic systems, and cause a disturbance in the flow of nerve impulses. This type of situation is considered to be a major precursor to the development of disease.

Because of inertial patterning, the functioning of the body's essential health-giving mechanisms becomes affected. If this stasis is resolved and natural motion restored, then the expression of intrinsic health can return. For example, a patient of mine who had been hit on the head by a cricket ball experienced months of depression. When the inertia held in his parietal bone was resolved, he described feeling as if a dark cloud had been lifted from him. In another case, a 5-year-old boy stopped wetting his bed when his slightly twisted sacrum started to express primary respiratory motion. A 28-year-old musician's digestive problems disappeared when the restriction in his diaphragm was treated. These are just a few illustrations of a principle which is seen at work every day in the treatment rooms of craniosacral practitioners.

UNITY OF THE BODY

In a real sense all life is inter-related. All men are caught in an inescapable network of mutuality, tied in a single garment of destiny. Whatever affects one directly affects all indirectly. I can never be what I ought to be until you are what you ought to be, and you can never be what you ought to be until I am what I ought to be. This is the inter-related structure of reality.[12]

REV. DR MARTIN LUTHER KING JR

Everything is connected

An important tenet of osteopathic practice is that the body functions as a totality in both health and disease. The different parts of the body often get separated for the purposes of study or examination, but in reality they are part of an interdependent system. When something is put under the microscope, it's easy to lose sight of the whole picture. In this way, it has become common practice in modern Western medicine to fragment the different aspects of a human being into separate areas. All parts of the body are seen to require the specialized attention of an expert in that particular organ or system (the cardiologist, gastroenterologist, urologist, etc.). Then, any psychological difficulties have to be dealt with by yet another specialist. Some patients end up seeing three or four specialists, with each one treating something different.

An organization

In actual fact, each part is directly connected to the whole and functions in relationship to all other parts. In this way, the body operates like a large organization such as a hotel.[13] In a hotel every employee is important, to ensure that everything runs smoothly and efficiently. The porters, managers, cleaners, cooks and receptionists are all necessary to keep things running. If any one job is not carried out, very soon it affects the functioning of the whole organization. Likewise in the body: if any part is disturbed, it can affect the functioning of the whole. As the physiologist Dr Irwin Korr observes, 'There is no such thing as a sick organ; there is only a sick man. Treating the part alone is not treating the man, while treating the man is to treat the part too.'[14]

Sophie's case

Sophie came for craniosacral treatment with a neck pain which had been getting steadily worse over the previous month, despite receiving physiotherapy treatment. She was an active and fit dancer in her mid-thirties, who was performing nightly in a West End London musical. However, her neck problem was starting to interfere with her ability to make any kind of physical exertion. This was making her feel irritable and frustrated with the limitations that she was experiencing. She reported that about six weeks previously she had twisted her ankle while rehearsing. As this was nothing very unusual, she hadn't paid it too much attention. However, she was still feeling some restriction in her foot, even though the initial swelling of her ankle had gone down.

On examination, I came to the conclusion that the ankle injury was probably still affecting the balance of movement in her whole body. Her pelvis was slightly twisted and, in turn, some rotation and stiffness had developed in her lumbar spine. This seemed to be creating a compensatory pattern in her neck.

During her treatment, we started working with the remaining inertia in her foot. From there it was possible to track the problems manifesting higher up in her body and encourage the expression of primary respiratory motion at each site of restriction. Within two treatments there was a great improvement in all her symptoms.

Sophie's case illustrates a simple point: if we do not look at the whole picture, we will likely miss the conditions which cause and maintain our symptoms. A Green Party slogan sums up this principle: 'Think globally, act locally.'

The whole person

Moreover, this law of unity applies to the whole person, not just our muscles and bones. The body is a part of a continuum – mind, body and spirit, and intelligently reflects the whole. Clearly, we are complex beings, with all our individual traits and unique experiences. Nevertheless, the body registers all of these experiences, thoughts and feelings, as well as more physical ones. Responses are accordingly created in the body's structure and functioning. For example, heart rate and breathing may change, muscles may contract or relax, or temperature changes may occur according to our situation. The patterning of the body becomes a distinctive expression of the totality of the individual. We probably have all become aware of this process at some point. How does your body reflect your current situation? What is it saying to you?

Finding wholeness

The primary respiratory system reflects the totality of the individual at the most fundamental level of physiological functioning. A clear and balanced expression of primary respiratory motion signifies the manifestation of health and integration involving the whole person. Where there is some fragmentation of our experience, this is reflected as a focal point of inertia. These are places where the Breath of Life is unable to find expression in the tissues. The essential purpose of craniosacral treatment is to help restore primary respiratory motion in areas of the body which have become fragmented in their connection to the whole.

As primary respiratory motion is restored, and fragmented parts of ourselves re-enter the flow of life, we become whole again. This is healing in its truest sense, for the word 'health' comes from the same Latin root as the word 'whole'.

Balanced alignment

Craniosacral treatment seeks the best possible conditions for the expression of primary respiratory motion. This is done by encouraging greater balance in the structure and function of the whole person. When this optimal alignment is found, it allows for fragmented areas to reconnect with their source of health. In this way, discordant parts of ourselves are brought back into focus. When thinking about this, I'm sometimes reminded of some old movies in which the dialogue never quite matches up to the movement on the actor's lips – the soundtrack is somehow out of synchronization with the pictures. If ever there's a time in the film when these two come back into alignment, there's always a feeling of great satisfaction![15]

INNER SOURCE OF HEALING

It is the primary role of the physician, whether the African witch doctor or the modern doctor, to entertain the patient while secretly waiting for nature to heal the disease.
ALBERT SCHWEITZER

Inner physician

A further principle of practice is that the body is a self-healing and self-regulating system. Essentially, all the capabilities and resources that we need for health and balance can be found within the body itself. While external remedies may *support* the emergence of health, they do not *create* it. Health cannot be administered from the outside.

The tendency of the body to repair itself and find balance is natural and innate; not something which has to be learned. This great intelligence is demonstrated in all the body's activities. For example, if we cut a finger, fluid congregates in the area, causing inflammation. This helps to isolate the region, preventing the spread of any infection. White blood cells, which are contained in the inflammatory fluid, automatically start to remove any toxins which enter. Clotting factors in the blood help to form a scab, and tissue repair follows. Without this extraordinary expertise, the body could not repair even the simplest cut. Dr Still referred to this intelligence as an 'inner physician' which is always there to encourage optimum health for the individual.[16]

Homeostasis

The cells of the body have a remarkable capacity to remain in balance. The various mechanisms which ensure this balance are another example of the body's prowess of self-regulation. This ability is called *homeostasis*. For cells to survive, the composition of the fluid that surrounds them needs to be constantly maintained in a state of equilibrium. Chemical balance, temperature and pressure are all factors which must be carefully regulated, or cells will suffer. This balance is maintained despite marked shifts in external conditions, such as changes in temperature, toxicity or oxygen, or from variations in our internal condition. The nervous and hormonal systems are constantly monitoring the body's physiology and then making appropriate adjustments. They do this by sending out compensatory chemicals, such as neuro-transmitters, endorphins and hormones. In whatever circumstances we may find ourselves, these mechanisms endeavour to maintain a physiological balance.

The pharmacist

As long as we are able to access the body's innate resources, health will follow. These resources are the tools of our 'inner physician'. Dr Still had the great insight that all the substances required to maintain health could be made available by freeing up their pathways of circulation. He wrote,

> All the remedies necessary to health exist in the human body. They can be
> administered by adjusting the body in such a manner that the remedies
> may naturally associate themselves together, hear the cries, and relieve the
> afflicted. I have never failed to find all the remedies in plain view on the
> front shelves and in the store house of the Infinite – the human body.[17]

Dr Sutherland pointed out that by facilitating primary respiratory motion, the practitioner becomes the pharmacist.[18]

Balance in our imbalances

At a fundamental level, all our self-healing and self-regulating capabilities are driven by the available potency of the Breath of Life. However, the capacity of this biodynamic potency can become overwhelmed by stressful experiences or trauma. This is when sickness results.

Nevertheless, in the event of sickness our body systems still intelligently seek balance. Our intrinsic biodynamic potency is still working, but it has to adapt. As far as possible in these circumstances, the body becomes organized so that any disease causes the minimum of damage. So, if cure is not possible, we develop compensatory patterns and find a balance within our imbalances.

Checks and balances

The manifestation of disease symptoms is part of this intelligent response of the body. If there is some imbalance in our lifestyle, such as too much stress, or a poor diet, the body lets us know by producing certain symptoms. These are like the red light flashing on a car dashboard, indicating that there is something going on that needs attention. If we are then able to deal with the origin of the problem, health will follow. If not, and we just carry on 'driving', the body's resources may be further tested. Symptoms can thus provide checks and balances to our excesses and deficiencies, pointing the way to a more harmonious way of living. In many ways symptoms are our friends ... by dealing with the circumstances that created them, we have an opportunity to find deeper levels of integration.

Intelligent responses

If we become sick, the body tries either to dissipate the illness or, if this is not possible, to contain it as best it can. The development of a fever to eliminate an accumulation of toxins, a protective tissue contraction in response to a trauma, or the containment of a malignant tumour to a particular location are all expressions of this intrinsic health. They are examples of the balancing power of nature in action. According to pioneering Naturopath Dr Henry Lindlahr, 'The science of natural living and healing shows clearly that what we call disease is primarily nature's effort to ... restore the normal functions of the body.'[19] Sickness can be seen as the best possible solution in the circumstances, and therefore an elementary expression of our wellness!

Working for the wisdom

Modern medicine's obsession to fight disease and eliminate its symptoms, without considering the underlying causes, reveals a basic mistrust of the intelligence of the body. Rather than fighting disease, the emphasis of the craniosacral approach is to support health. Our fundamental resource of health is the biodynamic potency of the Breath of Life. It is this potency which intelligently centres a disturbance to a particular location and contains any damage. If this intrinsic resource can be accessed and supported, then even more efficient expressions of wellness can emerge.

Craniosacral treatment works *with* the physiology of the body, not against it. The intelligence of symptoms is acknowledged, as well as the intelligence of the body's attempts to deal with them. However, in order to appreciate this, first we have to be prepared to listen to what the body is saying. Instead of fighting the body's wisdom, we may need to 'sit around a table' and hold some peace talks! Furthermore, this gentle and respectful approach obviates the risk of unwanted side-effects. Negative reactions to treatment are unlikely when the treatment simply supports the wisdom of the body.

Creating the conditions

The movement towards integration and health is a natural tendency, an ever-present and gentle force. A cut finger doesn't have to be told how to heal, but it does need to be kept clean and protected. This, at least, is the responsibility of the patient.

On some level, everything that we do (positive or negative) is in the pursuit of feeling well. Dr Becker once observed that, 'We fight – we live – in order to express health within ourselves.'[20] However, unfortunately, some of our attempts do not actually support the re-emergence of health. In fact, they often make matters worse. An asthmatic smoker whose immediate craving may be satisfied by another cigarette, is not necessarily going to get any better. Still, this may be the best that they can do at that time. However, the path to health necessitates developing the right conditions for the emergence of our intrinsic healing resources.

Health never stops

Life springs up wherever it has the opportunity: between the cracks of paving stones, in forests ravaged by fire or in disabled bodies and troubled minds. Health also is an irresistible force. There is never a time when our health-giving mechanisms are not working, for they are an intrinsic part of our lives. Even in more chronic or advanced cases of illness, the Breath of Life and our original intention of health are always present. By comparison, a log which has become jammed in a river may create turbulence in the water, but the river still flows on. Likewise, the Breath of Life still provides the organizing blueprint in an ailing body. The seeking of health never ceases. It is innate, intelligent and always there. In the words of Dr Becker,

The seeking of health from within is a continuous time, tissue, and tidal effort from conception to the final moments of physiological life. Within every trauma and/or disease entity, there is an effort on the part of body physiology to deliver health mechanisms through the local area of stress to full functioning health capacities.[21]

Moving on?

Chronic states of illness result when the mechanisms which help us to dissipate or adapt to stressful forces become overwhelmed.[22] If we cannot mount an effective response of adaptation, there is a tendency towards degeneration and death. However, this is still part of the natural intelligence of life. Recurrent cycles of birth, growth, decay and death can be seen everywhere in nature. Sooner or later the time will come for all of us to move on, and the river of life to take another course. Perhaps this is the ultimate adaptation.

Healing is not just about getting rid of symptoms, but about supporting and integrating individual wholeness.[23] Our wholeness is always available, whatever the circumstances. Someone who has cancer or AIDS can still be healthy. It is also possible to die healthily. As Dr James Jealous asserts,

Health ... is at the core of our being and cannot be increased or decreased to a greater or lesser degree. In other words, the health in our body cannot become diseased ... the health in the body actually transcends death. The health in our body is 100 per cent available 24 hours a day from conception until death, then it transpires. It does not expire.[24]

Margaret's story

Margaret was an 82-year-old neighbour whom I had treated on and off over many years for recurrent back pain. She had been ill with cancer for some time and was growing considerably weaker. She telephoned me because she was feeling very anxious about what was happening to her and wanted someone to talk to. When I went over to her house the next evening, Margaret immediately started to express her fear of death and what might follow. Would it be painful? What's on the other side? Every time she had tried to talk to her family about these things, they'd wanted to change the subject. Personally, I found her very refreshing in her honesty and need for answers.

At the end of our conversation I put my hands on Margaret's head to give her a craniosacral treatment. Within a short time her body started to relax, and she was able to let go of her worries. A beautiful experience of the long tide permeated through her body and a feeling of deep calmness entered the room. Two days later, I received a telephone call from Margaret's daughter to tell me that Margaret had died in her sleep that same night. When I look back, I consider that craniosacral session as one of the most profound treatments I have ever given.

Solution in the problem

In any diseased state, there is a potential for transformation. This potential is intrinsically and holographically contained within the disease itself. As acupuncturist Dianne Connelly puts it, 'Our struggle and our strength emerge from the same source, and (if) ... we were to follow either to the ends of being we would find ourselves at home.'[25] The same intelligent process which centres the disease can also be used in its cure. All that is required is a re-organization of the forces which underlie it.

As a parallel, this same principle is found in certain Buddhist meditation practices. In these meditations there is no attempt to get rid of negative tendencies, but to work *with* them in a gradual process of realization and transformation. By accessing the true nature of our problems they then become transformed into their fundamental, underlying qualities. For instance, hatred is thus seen as an unenlightened form of love. By realizing the essential love contained within the hatred, it is transformed. Hugh Milne points out, 'The chief characteristic of monsters in myths is that once they are faced, they wilt away, or even become allies (the forbidding wolf becomes the protective watchdog).'[26] Thus allegorical frogs can be transformed into princes, Sleeping Beauty into wakefulness, and Clark Kent into Superman!

Personal responsibility

Whatever therapeutic approaches we use, health cannot be imposed from the outside. Ultimately there is no wonder drug or wonder cure other than the intrinsic forces of nature. Healing is thus the prerogative of each individual. Therapies themselves cannot cure, but they can trigger and support a process of inner change. I firmly believe that I have never cured anybody in my life (apart from perhaps myself). My work as a therapist is simply to help create the conditions for the inherent potency of the patient to get to work ... the rest is up to nature.

Each of us should feel encouraged to take responsibility for our own health. However, from an early age we are taught that our bodies are like specialized pieces of machinery which we're not qualified to deal with.[27] In many ways we have become disempowered, giving all our responsibility to the doctor or therapist to 'make' us better. Consequently we may have forgotten how to listen to our body and follow its intrinsic wisdom. The process of taking responsibility may involve some re-education, in the truest meaning of the word. The word 'education' is derived from the Latin *educare*, which means 'to lead out' or 'to encourage that which is already inside'.

In an old Tibetan Buddhist wisdom tale, a woman asked her spiritual teacher, 'If these grand old living Buddha-teachers are as perfectly enlightened, awakened, omniscient, skilful, powerful and compassionate as we think they are, why don't they just wake us up from the sleep of delusion?'

'Who's asleep?', the master replied.[28]

Dealing with causes

While symptomatic relief is naturally a valuable goal of treatment, this should never be the sole focus. Any treatment which does not acknowledge the basic wisdom of the body risks the danger of suppressing symptoms, or of merely swapping one problem for another. This is akin to moving furniture around in a room. Things seem to have changed, but the basic living space hasn't – you're still living in the same room. Rearranging 'the furniture' will have little impact on the fundamental issues which underlie ill-health. However, according to the old adage, 'You pays your money and you takes your choice!'

Treatment from the inside

Dr Sutherland realized that the intrinsic potency within the patient's own body can be utilized for treatment, rather than having to apply any external forces.[29] Essentially, the craniosacral practitioner assists the body to make its own adjustments by encouraging a re-organization of its intrinsic healing forces. According to Franklyn Sills, 'This is an art of intelligent and intuitive listening.'[30] The therapist listens to the body's subtle physiological motions and any areas of restriction or inertia. Using the hands to reflect back to the body the pattern of inertia that it's holding, the therapist can facilitate the body's self-healing capabilities. The success of treatment is marked by a re-emergence of the Breath of Life in areas of disorder. In Chapter 7 we will look at some particular skills which are used to achieve this.

A *living process*

Everyone has their individual pattern of health, and so listening to the intelligence of the body requires individual attention. This also needs to be an open, fluid and dynamic process, because it works with the way in which the Breath of Life unfolds as a living expression. This involves a constant evaluation of primary respiratory motion with each patient and with each new moment, in order to follow how it wants to work. Just when you might think you understand the wisdom in the body, it can teach you more. Things are always changing, nothing stays the same – this is a feature of the rhythmic and dynamic nature of life.

5

PATTERNS OF
EXPERIENCE

---

*In order to cure the human body, it is necessary
to have a knowledge of the whole of things.*

HIPPOCRATES

FULCRUMS IN HEALTH AND DISEASE

*Since the goal of every patient is to return to normal, it is important that
the physician knows what is health functioning from within the patient
seeking his service.*[1]
DR ROLLIN BECKER

In this chapter we will look at the specific ways motion is organized, and what happens when
we encounter stresses which impact on the functioning of the primary respiratory system. An
emphasis will be placed on the underlying forces that determine how primary respiratory
motion is expressed. Some of the effects of inertia will also be considered.

Natural fulcrums

Any kind of motion is organized around a fulcrum; the still point around which things move.
Levers get their power to produce motion from their fulcrum points. In the body, craniosacral motion occurs around specific fulcrums which act as leverage points for the rhythmic movements expressed by different tissues. The potency that provides the power for
craniosacral motion is found at these fulcrum points, so they are always significant places for
the functioning of the body.[2]

Each aspect of the primary respiratory mechanism (bones, fluid, nerve tissue and membranes) has a *natural fulcrum* of motion. These are the places around which craniosacral
motion is expressed in optimum health. If there are no modifying or influencing forces present, motion is expressed with balance and symmetry around its natural fulcrums. The practitioner needs to be familiar with the natural fulcrums in the body, in order to discern normal
from abnormal functioning.

Embryology and the midline

The midline of the body has great significance for the organization of our growth, development and maintenance of health. The midline acts as a natural fulcrum around which all
aspects of primary respiratory motion are expressed. The organization of motion around the
midline can be seen in operation as far back as the time of early embryological development.
By about 15 days after conception, a line of cells, called the *notochord*, has formed along the
midline of the developing embryo. This pattern of growth along the midline is thought to be

determined by the ordering forces of the Breath of Life expressed within the fluids of the rapidly dividing cells.[3]

This midline orientating force has been called the *primal midline*.[4] The primal midline provides orientation and direction for cellular development. Without this midline axis, there is no sense of back/front, top/bottom or left/right.[5]

The notochord provides the axis of development for the central nervous system and vertebral column (see Figure 3.3, page 48). Once the growth of these tissues has been established, the notochord disappears.[6] Nevertheless, as more and more cells divide and other systems are formed, the primal midline remains the cardinal axis of embryological development.

The primal midline, in fact, remains as an organizing factor throughout our lives. The different tidal unfoldments of the Breath of Life are generated as radiances which are continually expressed along this midline (see Figure 5.1). From the subtle permeations of the long tide to the specific patterns of craniosacral motion, the midline acts as a place of orientation. According to Franklyn Sills, the primal midline becomes 'the main energetic and structural organizing axis of the human body ... The Breath of Life is continually arising along this axis throughout life.' He adds, 'In yoga theory it is the sushumna of the caduceus ... It is the reference beam of the hologram.'[7]

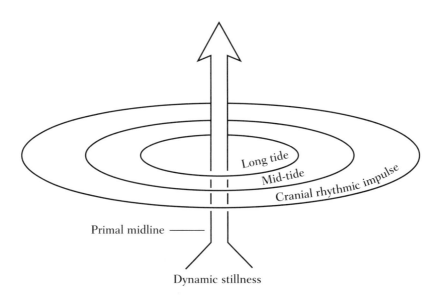

Figure 5.1: The three tides generated as radiances around the primal midline

Natural balance

As our body systems develop, all the different organs and tissues grow according to a remarkably ordered design along particular pathways. The specific pattern of how these tissues are embryologically formed helps to determine the natural fulcrum of their craniosacral motion. As an example, the central nervous system grows around a midline point located at the front wall of the third ventricle of the brain (see Chapter 3). This fulcrum remains as the point around which the central nervous system naturally expresses its primary inhalation and exhalation throughout life.

The cranial bones have their natural fulcrum at the joint between the sphenoid bone and occiput, the spheno-basilar junction (see Figure 3.16, page 69). This place is at the heart of the development of the cartilaginous floor of the cranium. The natural fulcrum of the reciprocal tension membrane system (Sutherland's fulcrum) is located along the midline straight sinus (see Figure 3.11, page 60). This is the place where forces converge to form the dural membranes during their embryological development.

In an ideal state, the body is able to express its craniosacral motion around these natural fulcrums. When this occurs, it indicates that there is no resistance or inertia held in the tissues and the ordering principle of the Breath of Life can be optimally distributed. However, stressful experiences can shift this balance and affect the way our inherent health is able to manifest. In this case, instead of craniosacral motion being organized around its natural fulcrums, other superimposed patterns develop.

Cellular contraction

Whenever faced with a stress or trauma, the primary physiological response of tissues is to contract. For example, if you are walking down the street and somebody knocks into you, you will naturally contract in response. This instinct helps you to protect and defend yourself. Even single cells can be observed under a microscope to contract when stimulated. However, once the stressful event has passed, cells and tissues naturally seek to release their contraction. Nevertheless, tissue contractions can remain if the body's intrinsic resources for repair and rebalancing are overwhelmed. In the biodynamic approach of craniosacral work there is a recognition of the underlying forces which control this process. We will now look in more detail at how these forces operate within us.

Biodynamic and biokinetic forces

The inherent ordering force in the body is the potency of the Breath of Life, our *biodynamic potency*. This 'organizes the cellular and tissue world', maintaining the health and balance of the body.[8] In its pure state, the expression of biodynamic potency is not conditioned by any of our experiences or stresses.

However, stress and trauma exert an influence on the functioning of the Breath of Life. Dr Becker referred to these stressors as *biokinetic potencies*.[9] They are the forces of our conditioning which may arise from factors such as physical injury, toxicity, infection, psychological, environmental or hereditary issues. These biokinetic potencies have to be compensated for by the biodynamic expressions of the Breath of Life. In this process, the natural balance of biodynamic potency becomes disturbed. Thus the terms 'biodynamic' and 'biokinetic' are used to describe an interplay of forces which occurs as our intrinsic health has to meet with any conditioning influences.

Inertial fulcrums

Any added force which affects the body, such as a blow, a fall or even a difficult emotion, carries with it a particular amount of energy: its biokinetic potency. When such stressful influences are encountered, there is natural effort on behalf of the body to seek optimal balance. In an ideal state, the body's intrinsic biodynamic forces are able to dissipate the impact of any biokinetic experiences. However, if the stress is very strong (or repetitive), the capacity of the body's biodynamic potency may be overwhelmed. The biokinetic force then remains within the body, carried around as 'extra baggage'.

When we are unable to dissipate biokinetic forces, the next best thing occurs: the biodynamic forces of the body centre them to a particular place in order to minimize the damage. Such a place becomes a site of inertia, and is referred to as an *inertial fulcrum*. Inertial fulcrums (rather than natural fulcrums) then become the points around which primary respiratory motion is organized.

Trapped potency

Substantial amounts of biodynamic potency may be required in order to centre biokinetic forces to particular locations. This biodynamic potency, which otherwise would be freely moving, becomes inertial along with the biokinetic forces it encloses. As a result, sites of

trapped potency and stasis are created. Within the core of, and maintaining every inertial fulcrum, are these *inertial potencies*. This concentration of inertial potency may be palpated by
the practitioner as a site of densification which affects the balance of primary respiratory
motion.

Disturbances of motion

Remember that tissues and fluids become organized in relationship to the forces which control their function. Where inertial potencies are present, the physiological functioning of the
body follows their direction. This is how patterns of resistance, contraction and disease are
created. In this way, stressful experiences which we are unable to resolve become woven into
the fabric of our tissues. These resistances are sometimes referred to as *osteopathic lesions* or
sites of *somatic dysfunction*.

Inertial fulcrums alter the way in which primary respiratory motion is expressed around its
midline axis and natural fulcrums. Instead, aberated patterns of motion are created. When
this happens in our own system, we will probably feel 'off centre'. As Franklyn Sills writes,
'The cellular and tissue world, rather than orienting to the blueprint of health alone, now
has to orient to the stress being centred.'[10] Dr Michael Shea describes,

> *The new fulcrum will have a new quality of movement that is distinctly*
> *different from flexion-extension of the midline bones and membranes or*
> *internal-external rotation of the lateral bones of the head. This aberated*
> *movement pattern will none the less have its own regularity and*
> *suspended fulcrum.*[11]

Eye of the storm

An inertial fulcrum is like the eye of a hurricane, which contains the power of the whole
storm.[12] A great deal of turbulence can result in the form of tissue and fluid fluctuations, contractions, pulls, twists and torsions. Thus, an inertial fulcrum is a place that itself is static, and
yet which contains the forces that organize patterns of disturbance. Significantly, the inertial
potency found within each inertial fulcrum is the essential factor at work at the heart of every
condition of ill-health. As Dr Becker observes, 'At the very core of every traumatic or disease
condition within the human body is a potency manifesting its interrelationship with the body
in trauma or disease.'[13]

Imprints of stress

The development of sites of inertial potency can start at the very beginning of life. Cells of the body may even retain the imprints of stressful experiences from the moment of conception.[14] As each new stress or trauma occurs, inertial fulcrums accumulate. If these fulcrums are not resolved, the tissues of the body take shape accordingly. In this way, the body retains the story of experiences which have significantly shaped our lives. As a result of unresolved inertial forces, events become held in the tissues like video tape. Furthermore, these tapes keep replaying whenever stimulated.

Secondary fulcrums

The intrinsic wisdom of the body always seeks optimal balance, given the prevailing conditions. Whenever inertial fulcrums are formed, other areas of the body may need to adapt to their presence. This produces secondary or compensatory responses. For example, if the lower back is fixed in a position of rotation to the right, the neck may need to rotate to the left for a balance to be maintained throughout the body. This capacity of the body to adapt is an important feature in maintaining health. Thus, a *primary fulcrum* may produce compensatory *secondary fulcrums*. Through the unity of the body, various inertial fulcrums may be held in relationship to each other.

Previous experience

Exactly how the body responds to new events or experiences is largely determined by what has gone before. As substantial amounts of energy are required to maintain patterns of inertia, over time the availability of biodynamic potency in the body can become lowered. Each new overwhelming experience may diminish the amount of vitality that is available to deal with the next. As a result, someone who is already traumatized, retaining deeply-held or numerous inertial fulcrums, may reach a point of 'overwhelm' after perhaps only a minor new stress or stimulus. Therefore, the presence of unresolved stresses provides a fertile ground for new ones to accumulate. It becomes much easier to be 'kicked' when you're already down.

Relative and the absolute

The interplay between our intrinsic biodynamic and added biokinetic forces determines the patterning and shapes adopted by the body. Essentially, this is an interplay between the relative and the absolute in our lives. The Breath of Life is a universal principle which flows through us – not a function of our personal experiences or individual characteristics. The great poet Rumi described this truth when he wrote:

> *Soul with a hundred thousand bodies*
> *Everything's myself; I talk only of me.*
> *Like a wave I rise in my own body –*
> *Sea and wave the same wild water.*[15]

In a state of ideal health, the functioning of our cells and tissues is in harmony with the universal principle of the Breath of Life. However, stressful experiences that become fixed by inertia will, to a greater or lesser degree, influence our ability to operate in accord with this universal principle. As Franklyn Sills explains,

> *Organization is always twofold. There is the universal within us, the*
> *Breath of Life and its potency. The cellular and tissue world naturally*
> *organizes to this universal as does the mind when it is still. Then there are*
> *the forces of our experience. The cellular and tissue world must also*
> *organize relative to its experience and potencies will respond. On the level*
> *of the mind, mental forms and self constructs are generated, on the*
> *emotional level, emotional affects are held and on the tissue level,*
> *inertia is created.*[16]

INERTIAL PATTERNS

> *Think of the body as a begging bowl for the spirit. When spirit is removed*
> *from the body, it is no longer inspired. And since spirit is the catalyst that*
> *keeps all things moving, the body without it falls into a deep state of*
> *inertia. Emotions no longer move fluidly; neither do thoughts and*
> *muscles. Everything is constipated.*[17]
> GABRIELLE ROTH

The way in which our bodies become structurally patterned is a unique expression of our health, history and experience. Patterns of inertia reflect the ways in which we hold ourselves in the world, revealing how we have become conditioned by our life experiences. A stiff neck, abdominal tension or back pain may be the outer evidence of this conditioning process. These *patterns of experience* are held in the tissues, fluids and potencies of the body, and organized around inertial fulcrums. As these patterns develop, our options for movement and choice become lost, reflecting the fixed positions we may have adopted for self-regulation, protection and balance.

Form, movement and quality

A pattern of experience has three main aspects: *form*, *movement* and *quality*.[18] Its 'form' describes the particular shape of the pattern. This is its structure or architecture. For example, a membrane or bone may be held in a twisted or rotated shape. It is likely that this will put a strain on associated tissues, which also become part of the form of the pattern.

A pattern's 'movement' is the particular way in which the tissues involved are able to express motion. Even though inertia is present, tissues holding a pattern of experience are rarely completely fixed or immobile. They can still express some kind of motion, albeit compromised. The movement of a pattern (i.e. its function) is in a reciprocal relationship with its form (i.e. its structure).

The 'quality' of an inertial pattern refers to its individual characteristics, tones and nuances. For example, tissues and fluids may exhibit qualities such as hardness or softness, lightness or darkness, strength or weakness. Other qualities include potency or dullness, flow, chaos, hesitancy, stillness, cold, heat, damp or dryness, etc. The pattern may even suggest colours or images such as a cold, grey February morning or sticky chewing gum (I've felt both of these!). A pattern may also evoke particular emotions and sensations with which it became associated at its formation. These are the individual traits which make the pattern unique according to the specific experiences held within it. Each aspect of a pattern (form, movement and quality) can be identified by the practitioner's sensory perception operating through his 'thinking, knowing, seeing fingers'.[19]

Direction of preference

Every pattern of experience is organized around a specific inertial fulcrum, which holds it in place and determines its possible options of motion. As mentioned, rather than being

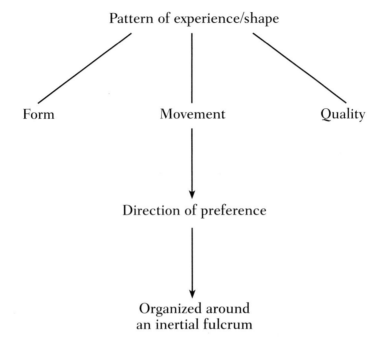

Figure 5.2: Pattern of experience

completely immobile, a pattern can nearly always express some motion around its organizing fulcrum. The particular way that it can still move is called its *direction of preference* (see Figure 5.2). For example, the motion of a cranial bone may be restricted in extension, but be free in flexion: its direction of preference. Where there are inertial fulcrums, motion occurs along specific, preset and often rigid pathways, narrowing the field of what is possible for that region. This can significantly effect the ability of tissues to express their intrinsic health.

Critical places

Inertial fulcrums are the critical places which maintain the shapes and patterns held in the body. It is here at the inertial fulcrum that changes must take place if healing is going to occur. This brings us to another central point in this work: *all true healing occurs at the organizing inertial fulcrum and not in the tissue patterns which develop around the fulcrum.* This fact can be easily overlooked. If only symptom patterns are followed, then we may miss the key factors which organize them.

If the trapped potency held at an inertial fulcrum is liberated, the Breath of Life can again permeate the tissues. This re-establishes a connection with the 'original matrix' in the area of disorder, and health is the result. As inertia is resolved, the expression of craniosacral motion around its natural fulcrums becomes restored.

Original intention

The ever-present original matrix is our original intention of health and an embryological imperative for order and balance. Put another way, it is our (pre-) birthright for health, which has been there since the very beginning of life. If there were no inertial fulcrums, there would be only an expression of this original intention, marked by a harmonious and balanced expression of the Breath of Life through all its unfoldments. To quote Dr James Jealous, 'What would happen if you claimed your original form? Wouldn't it be interesting to know who you were? Wouldn't it be interesting to know the intention of the Breath of Life when it made you?'[20]

EFFECTS OF INERTIA

Many sensations come, many thoughts or images arise, but they are just waves of your own mind. Nothing comes from outside your mind ...
Nothing outside yourself can cause any trouble. You yourself make the waves in your mind ... even though waves arise, the essence of your mind is pure; it is just like clear water with a few waves. Actually water always has waves. Waves are the practice of water. To speak of waves apart from water or water apart from waves is a delusion. Water and waves are one ...
a mind with waves in it is not a disturbed mind, but actually an amplified one ... our experiences are nothing but a continuous or repeated unfolding ...[21]
S. SUZUKI

Inertial fulcrums may become centred anywhere in the body – bone, membrane, nerve tissue or fluid. Organs, muscles and other connective tissues may also retain inertia as a result of stressful experiences. Some common problems which result from inertial patterns affecting the motion of cerebrospinal fluid and the central nervous system are summarized below. This summary is intended to give some examples of the applications of craniosacral work, but should not be interpreted as a prescriptive guide to the treatment of certain conditions.

River of life

Cerebrospinal fluid (C.S.F.), the 'great river of life',[22] is considered to be the primary point of contact between the potency of the Breath of Life and its expression in the body. It was perhaps for this reason that Dr Still perceived it to be 'the highest known element in the body'.[23] Any disturbance in the longitudinal fluctuation of C.S.F. can affect its ability to convey the inherent healing potency of the Breath of Life. Such disturbances may arise due to inertial fulcrums in any of the mechanisms that produce, distribute or reabsorb C.S.F. (see also Chapter 3).

Inertia held in the interconnecting system of ventricles in the brain may upset the production and potentization of C.S.F. Therefore, by facilitating the unobstructed motion of C.S.F. through the ventricles, the practitioner can help this vital fluid to potentize with the Breath of Life. This supports the functioning of all the important nerve centres and glands with which C.S.F. comes into contact.

After C.S.F. has circulated around the central nervous system, it is reabsorbed into venous sinuses and then drained back into the general circulation of blood. Many of the venous sinuses are formed within the folds of dural membrane that make up the reciprocal tension membrane system. Therefore, any pressure exerted on the dural membranes can create 'kinks in the hosepipe', affecting the drainage of fluid from the cranium.

A blockage within the venous sinus system can create a back-pressure of cranial fluid, leading to congestion. This may be palpated as a sense of stagnation in the fluids and heavy-headedness. Symptoms such as congestive headaches and a lack of energy may result, as the distribution of potency around the body becomes hindered.

Nervous system

Inertial fulcrums in the central nervous system affect the natural balance of its motility, and so influence its function. Due to the great complexities of the central nervous system, many kinds of disorders can result. Depending on the location of inertia, physiological functions such as lung respiration, appetite, digestion, circulation, co-ordination, movement and balance can be affected.

Inertia involving the central nervous system is often the result of compressive forces being exerted from its surrounding tissues, i.e. the cranial bones and reciprocal tension membranes. The cranial bones and membranes form the container for the brain, governing the space in which it moves, grows, develops and functions. Therefore, restrictions of motion involving these tissues may also impinge on the functioning of the brain and ventricles.[24]

Nerve facilitation

One important source of disturbance for the central nervous system is nerve *facilitation*. As this is such a common occurrence, it warrants being looked at in a little more detail. In this context the word 'facilitation' should not be confused with a state of ease or comfort. In fact, it refers to the ease with which a *problem* can start. Nerve facilitation refers to the excessive firing of impulses along a nerve pathway. This can lead to the irritation of whole regions of the nervous system.

Nerve cells communicate with each other by means of electrical impulses. These impulses are produced in response to some kind of stimulation, for example by pressure, heat or chemicals. A stimulus has to be sufficiently strong for an impulse to be conducted along the

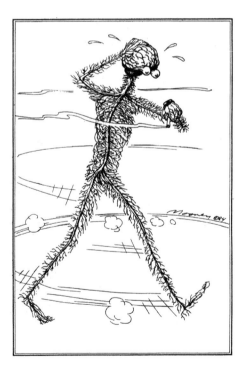

Figure 5.3: The Nervous System (cartoon © Gerry Mooney/Toonsmith Inc)

whole length of a nerve cell, or nothing happens at all. In other words, a certain threshold of stimulation needs to be reached for a nerve to conduct its impulse. Nerve cells do not conduct impulses along only part of their length. This is called the *all-or-none principle*.

Facilitated segment

If a nerve is already stimulated (for example, due to its compression), the threshold required for it to conduct an impulse can become lowered. Spinal nerves are often affected in this way, caused by the pressure that can result from restrictions involving the vertebrae (see Figure 5.4). Let's say that as a result of a back injury, nerve impulses become stimulated along the *sensory nerves* running from the vertebrae to the spinal cord. If the effects of this injury are unresolved, the nerves may remain in a state of constant irritation. As the threshold required for them to conduct impulses is lowered, they become prone to over-activity. This may cause a bombardment of irritable impulses sent to the spinal cord. As a result, the threshold required for the spinal cord to conduct nerve impulses may also be lowered.

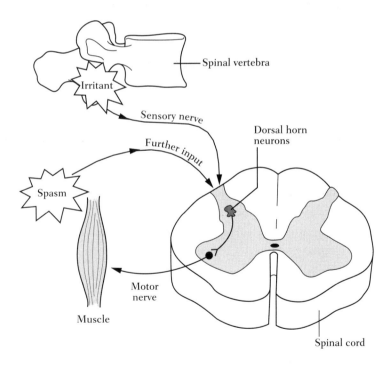

Figure 5.4: Facilitated segment

A *facilitated segment* is a highly excitable segment of the spinal cord which fires an abnormal degree of impulses. Due to the presence of a facilitated segment, irritable impulses are sent to the muscles, joints and organs that receive their *motor nerve* supply from that region of the spinal cord. This often causes the vertebrae and their surrounding muscles to become further restricted in their motion. Further irritable impulses from these bones and muscles are then sent back to the spinal cord, via the sensory nerves. In this way, a vicious cycle of irritation and over-excitability is created.

Effect on organs

The effects of a facilitated segment on the internal organs of the body can be significant. For instance, the stomach receives its *sympathetic nerve* supply from the mid-thoracic region of the spinal cord. If this region becomes facilitated, irritable nerve impulses may then be sent to the stomach. This is called a *somato-visceral reflex*. It can result in digestive sensitivities, or the person becoming prone to problems such as indigestion, inflammation, bloating or even ulcers. Breathing difficulties, heart problems, urinary and reproductive disorders, plus a wide range of other symptoms may result from facilitation of other regions of the spinal cord (see Figure 5.5).

Viscero-somatic reflex

However, the origin of a facilitated segment may be found in a diseased organ. For example, problems with the stomach, liver, lungs or heart may cause irritable nerve impulses to be relayed back to the spinal cord, causing its facilitation. This is called a *viscero-somatic reflex*.

Thus, a somato-visceral reflex is where a disturbance in the bones and tissues around the spine causes the irritation of an organ, while a viscero-somatic reflex is where the irritation originates in an organ, causing a disturbance at the spine. Facilitated segments explain why many problems affecting the internal organs improve once inertia at the spine has been resolved. When the source of spinal nerve irritation has been removed, the vicious cycle of facilitation is broken.

Spread of facilitation

Furthermore, facilitation of the spinal cord can spread up or down, creating whole regions of the central nervous system which become irritated. This irritation may extend all the way up to the brain stem, producing a condition where the whole nervous system becomes held in a

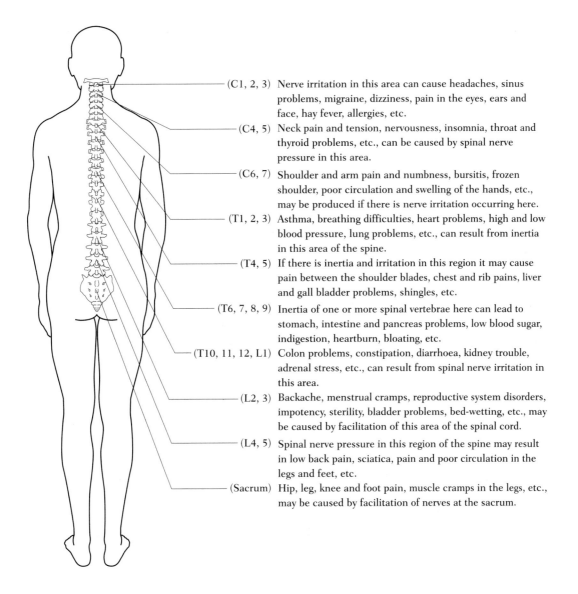

(C1, 2, 3) Nerve irritation in this area can cause headaches, sinus problems, migraine, dizziness, pain in the eyes, ears and face, hay fever, allergies, etc.

(C4, 5) Neck pain and tension, nervousness, insomnia, throat and thyroid problems, etc., can be caused by spinal nerve pressure in this area.

(C6, 7) Shoulder and arm pain and numbness, bursitis, frozen shoulder, poor circulation and swelling of the hands, etc., may be produced if there is nerve irritation occurring here.

(T1, 2, 3) Asthma, breathing difficulties, heart problems, high and low blood pressure, lung problems, etc., can result from inertia in this area of the spine.

(T4, 5) If there is inertia and irritation in this region it may cause pain between the shoulder blades, chest and rib pains, liver and gall bladder problems, shingles, etc.

(T6, 7, 8, 9) Inertia of one or more spinal vertebrae here can lead to stomach, intestine and pancreas problems, low blood sugar, indigestion, heartburn, bloating, etc.

(T10, 11, 12, L1) Colon problems, constipation, diarrhoea, kidney trouble, adrenal stress, etc., can result from spinal nerve irritation in this area.

(L2, 3) Backache, menstrual cramps, reproductive system disorders, impotency, sterility, bladder problems, bed-wetting, etc., may be caused by facilitation of this area of the spinal cord.

(L4, 5) Spinal nerve pressure in this region of the spine may result in low back pain, sciatica, pain and poor circulation in the legs and feet, etc.

(Sacrum) Hip, leg, knee and foot pain, muscle cramps in the legs, etc., may be caused by facilitation of nerves at the sacrum.

Figure 5.5: The effects of spinal nerve irritation

state of hypersensitivity and alert. In these instances, almost any kind of stimulus is experienced as pain or produces an exacerbation of other symptoms.

Facilitated segments are an important type of inertial fulcrum which has vast repercussions on total body physiology and health. They provide a link between the functioning of the musculo-skeletal system and the internal organs. They also point to the importance of a freely-movable spine for the maintenance of health.

Nerve disturbance

Epilepsy is a condition which is marked by an abnormality in the electrical discharge of the brain, frequently affecting the temporal lobe. It is often related to a disturbance in the natural motility of nerves in the temporal lobe and their consequent disorganization. Other conditions such as dyslexia, learning difficulties, attention deficit disorder (A.D.D.), mental illness and hyperactivity may also have their origin in inertial patterns which restrict the functioning of the central nervous system. For example, many practitioners have noted a correspondence between learning difficulties and compression of the occiput,[25] and with dyslexia and a restriction of the right temporal bone.

In these cases, treatment essentially involves working with the inertial fulcrums at the heart of the disturbance, thereby helping take the pressure off nerves that have become irritated. The key to resolving these issues is to restore the expression of the ordering principle of the Breath of Life in the central nervous system. The patient can then access the resources necessary to revitalize the nervous system and dissipate any trauma it holds.

Cranial nerves

There are 12 pairs of cranial nerves that emerge from the base of the brain. These nerves have important functions relating to the special senses (i.e. hearing, taste, sight and smell). They also control many muscles and glands of the face, head and neck. Furthermore, the widely influential vagus nerves ('vagus' literally means 'wandering') pass down through the body to regulate the function of the throat, heart, lungs and almost the entire digestive system.

Inertial fulcrums located in the bones, tissues and membranes of the head can produce facilitation of the cranial nerves. For example, tinnitus and hearing difficulties may result from the irritation of nerves that supply the ear. When pressure is taken off these nerves, these symptoms can greatly improve. Similarly, visual disturbances may result from inertial fulcrums causing irritation of nerves that supply the eye. I've treated a number of cases of anosmia (loss of the sense of smell) in which craniosacral treatment of the ethmoid bone and the olfactory nerves which pass through it has produced beneficial results.

The jugular foramina, located either side at the base of the head, provide small openings for the passage of three pairs of cranial nerves to gain exit from the skull. These include the vagus nerves. If one of the vagus nerves becomes facilitated, the symptoms can be far-reaching. Nausea (often together with migraine headaches), abnormalities in heartbeat, respiratory or digestive problems commonly result. Frequently, irritation of the vagus nerve is involved in cases of colic affecting young babies (see also Chapter 10).

Other nerves which also pass through each jugular foramen supply muscles of the throat, the largest salivary gland, and muscles of the neck and shoulders. A simple procedure to help disengage the suture between the occiput and temporal bones containing the jugular foramen can bring about fast relief for a wide range of symptoms.

Listening to your body

Take a few minutes to listen to the story of your own body. One way to help you to do this is to watch your breathing.

Sit quietly with your back comfortably supported, and start to bring your attention to the sensations in your body. Notice how you are breathing, but don't try to change anything. As you breathe in and out, become aware of the sensations and feeling tones that are being generated. Just acknowledge what is there. Scan your body from top to bottom. Perhaps there are some areas where you feel comfort and others where you feel discomfort. Maybe there is some heaviness or lightness, openness or contraction, fullness or congestion. You may notice pulsations, or places which feel either connected or disconnected. Get a sense of how your body has taken shape. What do these sensations tell you about yourself?

6

THE ART OF DIAGNOSIS

There is no need to run outside

For better seeing,

Nor to peer from a window. Rather abide

At the centre of your being ...

Search your heart and see ...

The way to do is to be.[1]

LAO TZU

ASPECTS OF DIAGNOSIS

*The core of this work is perceptual; the concept grew out of repeated
observation until the laws of nature became more clear. We learn to sense
the Whole. When one meets a patient one sees the Whole – a very rare
event in our modern world.*[2]
DR JAMES JEALOUS D.O.

Case history-taking, and especially the skills of palpation and perception, are the main diagnostic approaches used by craniosacral practitioners. These procedures focus on how health is being expressed within the patient and the location of any patterns of inertia. In this assessment an emphasis is placed on the motion, balance and qualities being expressed by the primary respiratory system.

Case history-taking

At the start of any treatment programme a case history is taken. This provides the practitioner with relevant details of the patient's current symptoms and medical history. Any history of trauma such as road accidents, surgery, difficult birth or dental work may be noted, as these can give vital clues to the source of a problem.

Details about family and social history, diet and psychological issues can also be useful, and may help to identify the patient's resources which are available to support the healing process. Medical tests such as X-rays, blood tests or scans may be recommended if further diagnostic clarification is needed.

Observation

The source of a problem may initially be indicated by the use of a keen sense of observation. When you see someone walking down the street, your first impression is often the most revealing. This is a skill that practitioners can develop to help them understand their patient's condition. For example, the way that someone walks in, sits down or holds themselves may enable the practitioner to notice what's going on. Their poise and balance may indicate how the tissues have become affected by stress or trauma. Does the patient move with ease, or do they have awkward and fragmented patterns of motion? How do they look? How do they speak? What is 'written' in their facial expression? What clues does this give about their condition?

Observing any asymmetries in the shape of the cranium or other parts of the body may indicate the presence of inertial patterns which have caused tissues to adopt structural changes. A postural inspection in either a standing, sitting or lying position can help to identify any problem areas. Particular attention can be given to the shape and balance of the spine, which acts as the central column of support for the body and has important consequences for our health (see Chapter 5, Facilitated Segments). Furthermore, the skin often reflects the balance of the body's internal processes, and so the identification of any marks or changes in skin texture can also help locate sites of inertia.

Palpation

The cardinal diagnostic approach in craniosacral work is to assess the subtle rhythmic motions produced by the Breath of Life. This is achieved through the faculties of palpation and perception. Palpation refers to the practitioner's ability to sense the patient's physiological patterns by impressions received through the fingers. This ability is dependent on the development of a finely tuned tactile sense. Both craniosacral diagnosis and treatment are accomplished through this faculty of touch, which needs to be both gentle and non-invasive in its application.

We will now consider some of the main elements that enable the practitioner to palpate the subtle realms of primary respiratory motion with a sense of clarity.

PREPARING THE GROUND

This we have now is not imagination.
This is not grief or joy.
Not a judging state, or an elation, or sadness.
Those things come and go.
This is the presence that doesn't.[3]
JELALUDDIN RUMI

Being present

The quality of the practitioner's presence is the starting point of any diagnostic enquiry and will also help to determine what results from treatment. Being present involves being open to all our aspects (physical, energetic and psychological), without any interest other than to appreciate how the body has become organized, and to facilitate its inherent health. Essentially, this practice includes an ability to 'be with' things. For example, we may need to be with another's pain, joy, grief, pleasure, anger or love. This can be a powerful therapeutic support if we are able to do this without seeking to hide or fix anything.[4] In addition, unless we are present for the health in another person, it is not actually possible to perceive and facilitate it.[5] In craniosacral diagnosis and treatment, the practitioner needs to be sufficiently 'in touch' and sensitive to the unique way that the Breath of Life organizes itself in each patient.

Turning up

The kind of presence which can provide therapeutic benefit is not a passive state. It involves the practitioner being prepared to engage in a clear and simple relationship with another, and requires the development of 'a keen and precise quality of attention'.[6] It means actually turning up! Like a finely tuned instrument, the practitioner has to be neither too loose nor too tight in this process. He needs to be able to sense subtle changes that are taking place in the patient's body, and to respond with fluidity. This is a dance between patient and practitioner, in which the Breath of Life within the patient is calling the tune.

Presence is perhaps one of the most challenging aspects in the practice of any of the healing arts, as most of us are so unused to paying attention with this degree of simplicity. Yet in many ways presence is the most natural thing in the world. When we are present we are able to meet someone with our 'is-ness' rather than our 'business'. Even though presence is at the foundation of good clinical practice, all too often doctors and therapists hide behind a plethora of techniques, protocols, projections and opinions (often protected by a large desk to sit behind), instead of simply being in the moment. Franklyn Sills observes that, 'Presence manifests as we allow our mind to still and rest wholly in the present. In stillness, it is possible to sense the presence of the deeper Intelligence at work within the human system.'[7]

Opinions

It seems that there are many things that can get in the way of being present. Dr Rollin Becker points out that, first, there are the opinions that the practitioner may have about the patient's condition. Then there are the opinions that the patient has about his or her own condition. Lastly, there is what is actually happening in the living physiology of the patient.[8] These three things do not necessarily coincide. In order to be present for the living physiology of the patient, it is necessary to let go of what we think we know and what we expect to find. Then, and perhaps only then, can we listen to what is actually there. Dr Sutherland noted that it is through this living experience that we can obtain *knowledge*, rather than mere information, about a patient's condition.[9]

Being and doing

A good quality of presence can, by itself, be an important factor in fostering the healing process. Perhaps many of us have experienced how an emergence of health can be triggered by this kind of support. As the psychotherapist Guggenbuhl-Craig observed, 'When two people meet, the totality of their psyches encounter each other; conscious and unconscious, spoken and unspoken, all have their effect upon the other.'[10] The implication here is that the results of treatment have, at least, as much to do with the practitioner's quality of *being* as with his *doing*.

Healing through resonance

To illustrate, on one occasion when working with a patient who was suffering from headaches and neck pain, I became aware of a jerkiness and unease which was palpable in his body. As I tuned in to his cranial rhythmic impulse, a sense of disturbance in the longitudinal fluctuation of cerebrospinal fluid became apparent. I noticed that this fluid motion was being expressed with various swirls and tremors. When I widened my field of perception to take in more of a whole sense of what was going on, I had the impression that there were thousands of tiny luminous 'energy molecules' which were chaotically bobbing around in his system. It was as if these 'molecules' didn't know what to do or where to go.

This patient confirmed that he was going through a very unsettling time. He was feeling the pressure of an important impending decision which could change the course of his life, but he had no idea of what to choose. I could feel his sense of anxiety and disturbance as it impacted against me, yet I remained calmly holding his head.

Within a short space of time I noticed how our two systems seemed to come into synchrony, as his cerebrospinal fluid fluctuation slowed right down and became much smoother. However, there was nothing that I actually did. It was as if the disturbance simply responded to my contact and was consequently able to settle. At this point, a sense of deep stillness emerged. When he stepped off the treatment table at the end of the session, he did so with a clear view of the right decision he needed to take. In this instance it was as if my contact simply provided his primary respiratory mechanism with a signpost; nature did the rest. This principle of healing through resonance seems to occur quite frequently in craniosacral work, especially when the practitioner is able to work from a place of inner stillness.

Pendulum clocks

This same principle is also observed in physics and in nature. Over 350 years ago, the developer of the pendulum clock, Christiaan Huygens, observed that pendulum clocks in the same place and with the same length pendulum have a tendency to move towards a synchronous motion.[11] Huygens also observed that there was a tendency for the heaviest pendulum to determine the frequency of others. Even if the heaviest pendulum was unable to fully influence the others, it would still partially draw the others' behaviour pattern towards its own.[12] According to osteopath Leon Chaitow, in biology 'One organism, or function, or cell, or dominant activity begins to "pull" or "drag" others towards its mode of behaviour.'[13] Chaitow compares a healthy, well-balanced therapist to a 'heavy pendulum' which can create a resonance that influences or 'pulls' the patient's state towards greater harmony.

In my own travels I've had the privilege and good fortune to study with some of the great contemporary Tibetan Buddhist teachers. One thing that I noticed early on was how easy it is to feel good when in their company. Some of these teachers have spent years in silent retreat and emanate such a feeling of calm, warmth and presence that you can't help being affected. A few years ago, one of the accomplished masters of this tradition was explaining to me that part of his practice is to see everybody he meets, young and old, rich and poor, as the Buddha. He explained, 'This is not putting something in which is not there, it is recognizing what we already really are, our fundamental nature.'[14] It was in that moment that I realized why it was so easy to feel good when in his company ... when he looked at you, he was seeing the Buddha! As Nelson Mandela commented in his presidential inaugural speech, 'As we become liberated from our own fear, our presence automatically liberates others. And as we let our own light shine, we unconsciously give other people permission to do the same.'[15]

Being centred

If we wish to help someone else find their health, we ourselves need to be in touch with a sense of our own balance and perspective. There are a number of ways which practitioners use to help them find this balance, but each person may have their own approach. Some practitioners take a few slow breaths to help them feel centred, or just sit quietly for a few moments prior to making physical contact. How this is done is not so important, but it is important to first find a clear ground from which to palpate and listen.

One approach commonly used by craniosacral practitioners to help them become centred is to establish what are called 'practitioner fulcrums'. As we have previously noted, a fulcrum is a place that orientates motion. A practitioner fulcrum is a reference point around which the therapist can orientate, so that he doesn't get lost in his listening. Simple visualizations can be used to help establish these reference points, so helping the practitioner feel grounded and enabling him to find a clear relationship with his patient. This skill is of great importance for craniosacral work ... and beyond. It is a life skill which can be used as a method for remembering who and where we are. My own experience is that if these fulcrum points are established it helps us to remain steady, even when turbulence is blowing all around.

Establishing practitioner fulcrums

Find a comfortable seated position and take a minute to place your attention on your spine. Imagine that there is a line which goes from the base of your spine (coccyx) to a point in the ground beneath you, as if your spinal cord continues down into the earth (see Figure 6.1). This line is like dropping an anchor into the earth from the base of your spine. It provides you with a reference point to the ground beneath you. Imagine that this anchor or fulcrum is also able to move, and so does not fix your position. Notice how it moves as you lean forwards and then backwards. As you lean forwards the fulcrum moves back in the ground, and as you lean backwards it moves forwards. The establishment of this fulcrum is often helpful if we are faced with confusing or powerful experiences. It gives us a relationship to the ground.

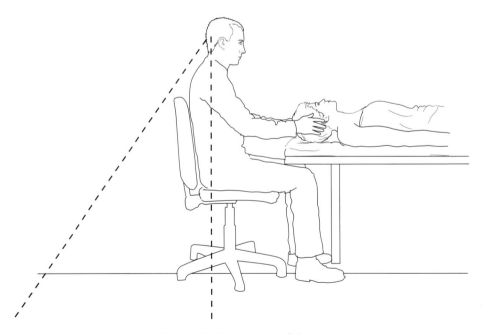

Figure 6.1: Practitioner fulcrums

Another useful fulcrum to establish is to imagine a line going from the back of your head diagonally down into the ground behind you (see Figure 6.1). This line is like a continuation of the angled straight sinus along which 'Sutherland's fulcrum' is located. Imagine that this line passes diagonally down into the ground at an angle of about 30 degrees from the external occipital protuberance, a centrally raised bump located at the back of the occipital bone. This is about an inch above the hollow where the top of the neck meets the skull.

This connection to the ground behind you helps to give an orientation between your front and back. It can provide the practitioner with a sense of the physical and energetic distance between himself and his patient. Again, it is a movable fulcrum. If you lean forwards and then backwards, you will notice how the angle of this line changes. An awareness of this fulcrum can help find the right balance in our own posture (and quality of intention) as we reach out to someone else. Furthermore, its establishment prevents the craniosacral practitioner from leaning too far into his patient. If this happens the patient's primary respiratory system may feel crowded. Alternatively, without paying attention to this fulcrum the practitioner's contact may be too remote or distant.

Some practitioners also find it helpful to establish fulcrums at their left and right sides by visualizing lines from the sides of their head going diagonally down into the ground at each side. These are like the guy ropes of a tent. Some also like to establish a 'sky fulcrum' by visualizing a line from the top of the head up into the sky above. This fulcrum can give an awareness of spaciousness above and around. Additionally, if the practitioner leans into his elbow contacts on the treatment table, these points can act as important fulcrums for his palpating hands.[16]

Getting orientated

An awareness of these fulcrum points can provide us with a sense of where we are, particularly if the boundaries between us and someone else are feeling confused. Due to the fact that a lot of craniosacral work is done while sitting still for many minutes at a time, it can be quite easy for the practitioner to 'space out' or get sleepy. At other times, if we encounter patterns of trauma and suffering (our own as well as someone else's), we may naturally be deeply affected. It's especially on these occasions that establishing these fulcrums is useful.

If at any stage during a treatment session the practitioner gets lost or blurred, he can remind himself of all or any of his fulcrums as a means of re-establishing orientation. When experienced in this process, it need not take more than just a few seconds.

When the practitioner is settled in his fulcrum points, it is then helpful to find a place in his own body from where he feels comfortable to listen. Such a place can act as 'an inner anchor',[17] enabling impressions from the physiology of the patient to be more easily registered. Some practitioners like to listen from the heart, others from the abdomen, and others from the head or throat. In this way, the practitioner's own body acts as a kind of barometer for any subtle changes taking place, and he can then begin the process of tracking the story of his patient's system.

Some people in the healing arts get worried by the idea of picking up 'negative energy' from others. However, by being centred in their own fulcrums any such problems become like 'water off a duck's back'.

Craniosacral contact

Physical contact may mean many different things to different people. It can be loaded with different implications according to how we have become conditioned.[18] For some, touch is threatening, bringing memories of trauma or abuse, for others it is reassuring and comforting, for others it may have sexual connotations. In this context the practitioner needs to have a light and spacious touch, a neutral intention (one which is not seeking anything or having any expectations) and a wide perceptual view (see Figure 6.2). These qualities enable the patient's body to unfold its story in a safe and supportive context. They also enhance palpatory sensitivity and the effectiveness of the therapeutic contact.

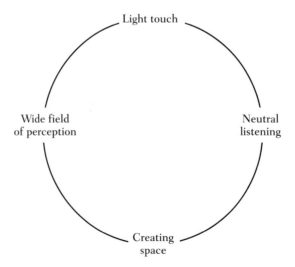

Figure 6.2: Craniosacral contact [19]

Light touch

Craniosacral work involves extremely gentle forms of contact. A lightness of touch is a prerequisite to be able to palpate the subtleties of primary respiratory motion. It is estimated that no more than 5 grams of pressure (about the weight of a dime or 5-pence piece) should be used.[20] This contact can be likened to a butterfly alighting on a leaf or how a water spider perches on the surface tension of water.[21] If the contact is too heavy, the sensitive mechanisms which express primary respiratory motion can 'shut down' in response to the compression exerted by the practitioner.

A lightness of contact 'invites the soul to swim up to the surface to meet the contacting fingers'.[22] However, conversely, a touch which is too light or remote is not sufficiently engaging to be able to feel anything, and may also trigger distress. Therefore, a delicate balance needs to be negotiated which enables the patient to feel comfortable and safe, and the practitioner to palpate the patient's physiology effectively. Each patient may require a particular quality and depth of touch, one that best suits their needs at that time.

Negotiating contact

Sometimes, parts of the body (e.g. the head, pelvis or abdomen) may be particularly sensitive to any kind of touch. Therefore, a slow negotiation of contact, made with a spacious intention, avoids creating any unnecessary awkwardness or discomfort. During this process particular attention can be paid to the subtle signals coming from the patient. These signals may be felt as a sense of the hands being pushed away, or the patient expressing a need for more space (either verbally or non-verbally). There may be certain stages when the practitioner may need to pause and keep his hands at a particular distance from the patient's body before moving any closer. In particular, if a patient is holding a lot of trauma this kind of sensitive negotiation is crucial. Otherwise, contact may be perceived as threatening or even abusive.

Boundaries

Well-defined boundaries between practitioner and patient are a necessity for providing clarity in the therapeutic relationship. However, the loss of these boundaries can easily occur when engaged in deep contact with another person. If we are not mindful of this fact we may become drawn too deeply into each other's issues. It is then impossible to 'see the wood for the trees'.

Touch is a powerful therapeutic tool, but for a depth of healing to occur this contact needs to be free from any agendas which may interfere with the natural processes of the patient. Personal needs, even an emotional need to help someone, can create a loss of boundaries and therefore a loss of clarity. When this occurs, confusion might arise about which sensations belong to the practitioner and which belong to the patient.[23] For example, 'Is what I'm feeling coming from you, or from me?' or 'Do I feel better/worse because of you or because of me?' This can be tiring and a hindrance to a feeling of safety and support during treatment.

Clear boundaries enable each person to appreciate what is truly their 'own' and be empowered to access healing from within. When the boundaries are clear, the practitioner can then maintain a sense of both himself and of his patient, so that any experiences in this relationship do not become blurred. However, boundaries should not become barriers. The presence of a truly caring and compassionate contact provides enormous benefit.

Practitioner neutral

The kind of mental state which is best suited to craniosacral palpation is sometimes referred to as the *practitioner neutral*. This is a neutral kind of listening, where there is an equanimity without a personal agenda. While this is an easy thing to say, it is not always an easy thing to practise, as we all can become clouded by our opinions, emotional needs and expectations. Therefore, this work necessitates a commitment by practitioners to work with their own projections, expectations and needs. This can prevent any personal issues of the practitioner from interfering with the natural therapeutic processes of the patient. As Dr John Upledger states, 'We therapists should always keep in mind the tremendous power that our intention, attitude and expectation have with the patient and their response to treatment.'[24] Craniosacral palpation is at its most precise and effective when practised without expectations. This involves an 'ability of the practitioner to reach out to the patient and meet them where they are, not where we would like them to be'.[25]

Expectations

There is a lovely story revealing some rich Jewish wisdom about letting go of expectations. This story is set in Czarist Russia during the early 1900s. During this time the local Jewish population was being persecuted, and many were forced to leave their homes in search of a new life. In one small village a rabbi used to walk across the village square on his way to pray at the synagogue; he'd been doing this at the same time each morning for at least 40 years.

One morning as the rabbi was making his way through the village some policemen were watching him from the steps of a police station which overlooked the square. They had had too much to drink the night before and were still somewhat 'hung over'. They decided to poke some fun at the rabbi. The policemen had seen the rabbi pass through the square every morning at the same time for as long as they could remember. However, this time one policeman shouted out in a mocking tone from the top of the steps, 'Hey! Rabbi, where are you going?' The rabbi turned around, looked up towards the policeman, shrugged his shoulders and replied, 'I don't know.'

This was not what the policeman expected to hear, so he shouted again, this time a little more forcefully, 'Rabbi, where are you going?' Again came the reply, 'I don't know.' This answer made the policeman frustrated because he saw that, as usual, the rabbi was making his way to the synagogue. He ran down the steps, took hold of the rabbi's collar and shook him, demanding, 'Where are you going?' The rabbi shrugged his shoulders and again replied, 'I don't know.' The policeman now became angry. He grabbed hold of the rabbi and dragged him towards the police station, arresting him for such insolence. At the top of the steps the rabbi turned to the policeman, saying 'You see, you never know!'[26]

Being at rest

In craniosacral work one may never quite know what really needs to happen for the patient, but the intelligence within the patient's own system does. The practitioner has to go along 'for the ride',[27] simply following and trusting the ordering principle of the Breath of Life and how it needs to work. Therefore, finding a neutral place from which to practise is of critical importance if the patient's self-healing forces are to be supported without interference.

Finding a 'practitioner neutral' involves developing a quality of attention which is able to be at rest.

Paradoxically, being at rest requires practice, as distractions and stimuli are all around. The spectre of violence grabs our attention on the nightly news, our emotional life becomes played out through the 'soaps', and battles rage to arouse us to buy things that promise happiness. However, the real problem with this bombardment is that we often lose sight of ourselves in the process. Our attention becomes habitually taken away from ourselves, so we become out of touch. We lose our own sense of being. We then often crave even more stimulation just to be able to feel anything at all.

Accessing a practitioner neutral means developing an attention which is neither being drawn away nor preoccupied with ourselves. It involves finding a place where our attention is neither coming nor going, but resting at a neutral point somewhere in between. The ability to find this place of stillness to listen from is another foundation of clear craniosacral palpation.

Beginner's mind

Being neutral also means listening with a sense of enquiry and wonder, as well as having no judgement or expectation of what may be found. It implies being with another person from a place of 'unknowing'. This may feel quite scary at first, as we let go of what we think we know and move into a deeper listening. This kind of attention is called 'beginner's mind' in Zen Buddhism.[28] It involves seeing things as if for the first time. As Confucius is quoted, 'He who departs from innocence, what does he come to?' Children have beginner's mind quite naturally, but as adults we're usually encouraged to lose it.

When I was about three years old, I had an imaginary friend whose name was 'Gog-gog'. One day I told my parents about how Gog-gog looked after me. He would appear at special times and take me on wonderful adventures. Sometimes, together, we would fly out of my bedroom window and circle around the garden and up over the neighbour's houses to look at the view. When I told my parents of this adventure, they laughed and I felt deeply hurt. I learned that Gog-gog was an object of ridicule and it was better not to speak about him. I put him out of my mind until many years later when, flicking through a book on Celtic mythology, I saw that the names of two ancient spirits who took care of small children in our area were called Gog and Magog. There are even two old trees in the east of England named after these great protectors of children.

Most of us are told to put away such childish perceptions, so that from an early age we learn to accept only those thoughts and feelings which comply to the prevalent world view (e.g. our parents' and teachers' views). We may consequently live out our lives within the conformity of a narrow but accepted range of perception. We may become intellectually smart, but lose the ability to trust in our instinctual 'felt sense'. However, this kind of intellectual knowing does not encompass the realm of our inner wisdom and is not enough to reconnect us with our source of health. In order truly to appreciate our deeper intelligence, we need to make a perceptual shift.

THE ART OF PALPATION

The wonder of touch is the wonder of human kindness.[29]
DIANNE M. CONNELLY

Language of the body

Anatomy is the language of the body. A good knowledge of anatomy enables the practitioner to understand the messages which the body communicates. Fluid, bone, membrane and nerve tissue each have their 'language', and convey their state of health in particular ways. Each of these can speak to the practitioner through the patterns and qualities of their primary respiratory motion.

A clear diagnosis is the springboard for effective treatment. Therefore, the practitioner needs to be able to recognize accurately how the body has become patterned by experiences, and to appreciate the forces which organize its motion. When treating, the practitioner's hands may need to reflect back the *specific* pattern that tissues are holding before they are ready to resolve their inertia. If a clear diagnosis is not established, then treatment can become a 'hit or miss' affair.

Finger sensitivity

Palpation can be defined as sensing with the hands. This is a process in which information is transmitted to the brain by sensory nerve endings in the fingers called proprioceptors. These nerve endings relay information about motion and position. The fingers contain the highest amount of nerve proprioceptors of any area of the body, making them acutely sensitive to even the most minute of impulses.

Figure 6.3 (page 136) depicts a homunculus. This is a diagrammatic representation of the proportional amount of the brain which is used to receive impulses from different regions of the body. The larger the area of the body in the drawing, the more 'brain space' is devoted to it. As indicated, a significant proportion of the brain is dedicated to the hands, making them probably the most sensitive parts of the body. They are far more receptive and responsive than any machine invented, distinguishing them as ideal instruments for feeling subtle movements and changes in the body.

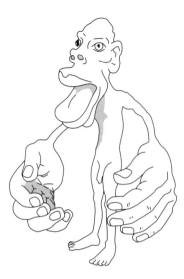

Figure 6.3: Sensory homunculus – the proportion of the brain used to process sensory information

According to Dr Harold Magoun, 'The human hand has been called the greatest single diagnostic instrument known to man. Marvellous as the advances of objective science may be, nothing takes the place of a searching analysis of the tissues with a well-trained palpatory sense, to determine not only the condition present but also the best procedure to modify or remedy it.'[30] Interestingly, some years ago an extremely sensitive instrument for measuring magnetic fields was invented, called the Superconducting Quantum Interference Device (or 'SQUID'). For the first time it became possible to measure the magnetic fields which surround the human body, and it was found that the hands have by far the highest field strength of any part of the body.[31]

Palpation of health

The hands in craniosacral work are used as 'perceptual antennae'.[32] The fingers learn 'how to feel, how to think, how to see' the patterns, qualities and nuances of primary respiratory motion.[33] The subtle rhythms of the Breath of Life are essentially expressions of wellness, carrying our original matrix of health into the body. Therefore, palpation of the primary respiratory system gives the practitioner direct access into the underlying condition of health and any restrictions to its expression. It also enables the practitioner to assess the body's available resources, which can be utilized in treatment.

Awareness with subtle senses

In addition to the faculty of touch, the physiological processes of a patient can sometimes make themselves known via a variety of other sensory impressions. For example it may be possible for a practitioner to 'see' a disturbance in the form of visual images. The way this information is received may be similar to how sonar waves permeate the ocean.[34] When an area of contraction or condensation is met, there is an echo back which can be registered by the sensory awareness of the practitioner.

It's not infrequent that the faculty of smell can give the practitioner valuable clinical information. There have been many occasions when I have smelled anaesthetic drugs emanating from a patient who was accessing 'tissue memories' of surgical trauma. Some practitioners report auditory perceptions, in which impressions about their patient are heard. It may be possible to hear the subtle 'buzz' being given off from someone who is in a state of nervous excitation, even though they are not speaking. It seems that all of our senses can be refined to pick up tones which are often outside of what is considered to be our normal range of perception. Furthermore, intuitive (sixth-sense) impressions can also be very revealing.

A few years ago a man in his early twenties came for treatment of a frozen shoulder. As soon as he walked in the room I had an awkward feeling about him, but didn't know exactly why. While I was taking his case history there was something shadowy in his manner which made me feel uncomfortable. This continued as I began the process of palpation. On his second visit, my awkward feeling was explained when he disclosed that he had been involved in terrorist activities. It became clear that he was still full of bitterness, justifying the use of violence for his cause. I started to think that perhaps his frozen shoulder was nature's way of preventing him from engaging in more violence. If this was the case, the last thing I wanted to do was to help free his shoulder. I had a deep sense that, in the circumstances, there was nothing I could do for him. I asked him to consider the messages that his own body was giving him and suggested that he let nature take its course for a while. Who knows where this kind of information comes from? Perhaps this case was just out of my league.

Tuning in

The start of every treatment session is marked by a time of tuning in, when the practitioner 'listens' through the fingers to the qualities of primary respiratory motion. Tuning in is usually done from the cranium, the sacrum or the feet, but can be practised from anywhere in the body.

Any disorder is marked by restrictions or distortions in the symmetry, quality, rate or amplitude of primary respiratory motion. This may manifest as a lack of motility and mobility in the tissues, a low potency or 'drive' in the fluids, and specific patterns of inertia. We will now consider some of these indications of physiological function.

Palpating the C.R.I.

Earlier (in Chapter 2) we practised an exercise to palpate the cranial rhythmic impulse in our own heads. We placed our hands gently on our cranial bones and focused attention on the movements of these 'corks floating on the tide'. We may have noticed the flexion/extension and external/internal rotation of the cranial bones as they express their reciprocal tension motion. In this way, we may have perceived motion patterns expressed at the level of the cranial rhythmic impulse (C.R.I.). Within the C.R.I., tissue and fluid rhythms can be experienced at an average rate of 8–12 cycles per minute.

Perception of this level of physiological functioning reveals how the tissues 'ride' on the deeper tides. Attention may be placed on the rhythmic motion of specific structures, such as a cranial bone or a membrane, or the motility of the central nervous system. The longitudinal fluctuation of cerebrospinal fluid can also be palpated to determine how this important carrier of potency is functioning.

Fluid drive

The quality of motion expressed by the longitudinal fluctuation of fluid is largely determined by the degree of potency it expresses. The strength or force of this motion is referred to as the system's *fluid drive*. If the underlying potency becomes diminished or restricted in its expression, then the fluid drive will be weaker. This may be felt as a sense of dullness, congestion or lack of 'spark' in the expression of longitudinal fluctuation. A weak fluid drive is indicative of deficient resources available for healing. Low potency affects the very foundations upon which our health is built and is often found in states of chronic illness or exhaustion. Therapeutically, the priority in these situations is to build up the availability of these vital healing reserves.

Amplitude

If the quality of fluid drive is reduced, or if inertial fulcrums create restrictions, the degree of motion expressed by tissues can be diminished. A cranial bone, for example, may be able to express its craniosacral motion in all the normal directions, but only moves within a very small range. This range is called its *amplitude*.

Some practitioners also place an emphasis on measuring the rate at which tissues express their craniosacral motion. This rate can vary according to circumstances, and so may provide an indication of physiological changes taking place. However, my own experience is that measuring the rate provides less valuable clinical information. The rate gives a number (i.e. so many cycles per minute), but the qualities of fluid drive and amplitude point to the available potency in the system, which can be important for both diagnosis and cure.

Palpation of inertia

If the body is holding patterns of resistance, the midline structures may not be able to express their natural craniosacral motion of flexion/extension, and the paired structures may be inhibited from expressing their external/internal rotation. Motility, the inner breathing of tissues, may also be lost.

When palpating at the level of the C.R.I., inertia is perceived as particular tissue restrictions organized around an inertial fulcrum. These inertial patterns may be palpated as a loss of tissue mobility, resistances, adhesions, compressions, pulls, asymmetries, fluid congestion and lateral fluctuations of fluid. All of these indicate some form of stressful experience which has become held in the body, producing a conditioned pattern of craniosacral motion away from its natural fulcrums.

It is important for the practitioner to ascertain the site of the inertial fulcrum which is at the heart of a particular pattern. This is done by noticing the still or stuck place around which the pattern has become organized. This place is like the 'eye of the hurricane', containing the whole potency of the storm.[35] It is at the inertial fulcrum that the key is found which can unlock the forces maintaining the pattern.

Lateral fluctuation

If the longitudinal fluctuation of cerebrospinal fluid meets the resistance provided by an inertial fulcrum, various eccentric patterns of fluid motion are produced. This resistance is like a rock on a smooth, sandy beach. Instead of the water being able to gently glide up the beach, all kinds of swirling motions are created as it hits the rock. These *lateral fluctuations* of fluid may be palpated in the body in the form of eddies, currents, whirlpools or congestion.

When the practitioner notices any movement of fluid which is not expressed as a natural longitudinal fluctuation, it is indicative of resistance in the system. If there is no resistance present, the longitudinal tidal motion of fluid is smooth and even, and carries a good quality of fluid drive. Noticing the places around which lateral fluctuations of fluid are produced can provide the practitioner with a clear sense of where inertial fulcrums are located.

Shutdown

If the resources of a person's primary respiratory system become overwhelmed, their cranial rhythmic impulse can temporarily stop. This is called a *shutdown*. It is a self-protective physiological reaction, marked by an abrupt and sudden cessation of rhythmic motion. Dr John Upledger has named these phenomena 'significance detectors', because they indicate that a significant experience for the patient has been accessed.[36] They reveal the presence of some kind of physical and/or emotional distress held in the tissues, often occurring when the body is in the same position that it was at the time of receiving a trauma. Shutdowns indicate that, for the time being, the patient is unable to access the resources to deal with the experience which has been evoked.

It's worth noting here that a shutdown differs from another phenomenon called a *stillpoint*, which occurs in states of deep physiological rest (see Chapter 7). While both a shutdown and a stillpoint involve a cessation of the cranial rhythmic impulse, they have very different qualities. During a stillpoint there is a smooth and gentle settling of the rhythm as it relaxes into stillness. In a shutdown, motion comes to a screeching halt.[37]

'CONVERSATION' SKILLS

To work with living mechanisms in a living body,
we need living palpatory skills.[38]
DR ROLLIN BECKER D.O.

Asking questions

Craniosacral work is essentially a practice of listening to and facilitating patterns of primary respiratory motion. However, it is also possible to 'talk' to the body by engaging it in a 'conversation' to clarify its story. The practitioner can ask questions through his fingers, and then listen to the responses. In this way the body can 'talk back', letting the practitioner know of its priorities. The perceptual focus of the practitioner, and how he meets a patient's system, determine exactly what can be palpated. As Dr John Upledger remarks, 'What you "know" seems related to which questions you have in mind during examination.'[39] Tissues can be engaged in particular 'conversations' by the practitioner bringing specific enquiries into his hands during palpation. This is done by introducing subtle suggestions through the fingers.

Motion testing

For example, it's possible to check if a particular bone prefers to express flexion or extension. At the start of a flexion phase of craniosacral motion, a subtle encouragement for the bone to move into flexion can be made through the practitioner's hands. How the bone takes up that suggestion is then noted. To test for extension, a subtle encouragement can be suggested at the start of an extension phase. If the bone moves into one phase of craniosacral motion more easily than another (or if there is some other asymmetry), it indicates the presence of inertia. If the bone moves into flexion, but doesn't move so easily into extension, then it is holding what is called a 'flexion pattern'. Inertial patterns are named after their preferred direction of motion. Therefore, a flexion pattern describes tissues which are stuck in flexion and so cannot move into extension.

Engaging the body in a 'conversation' to clarify how it holds patterns of experience involves a clarity of questioning and an ability to listen to its responses. This kind of enquiry is traditionally called *motion testing*. Like all approaches in craniosacral work, motion testing is done with gentleness, spaciousness and a respect for the boundaries of the patient's system.

Dialogue with fluids

Earlier, we noted that inertia creates eccentric patterns of motion in the fluids, called lateral fluctuations. Observing how the fluids move around a pattern of resistance can indicate the location of the organizing inertial fulcrum. If any clarification is needed, subtle suggestions of motion can be introduced into the fluids to reveal how they behave. The practitioner can suggest a gentle push into any lateral fluctuations with his hands, which are placed either side of the part of the body being assessed. This is like softly pushing a swing into the direction it is moving, thereby helping to intensify or amplify its motion. Furthermore, if lateral fluctuations are not already obvious, they can be gently initiated. This is done by the practitioner subtly intending a push into the fluids from one hand to the other hand, and then back again.

Tracking how the practitioner's suggestion is taken up by the fluids can pinpoint the inertial fulcrum. For example, do the fluids echo back or become absorbed in the tissues? If the fluids encounter a site of inertia, they will bounce back as they hit the tissue resistance, creating a rebound effect which can be felt by the practitioner's suggesting hand. Watching for the place around which any lateral fluctuations, such as eddies or currents, are produced helps to confirm the location of the inertial fulcrum.

Rachel's story

Rachel, a woman in her late twenties, came for treatment of an acute lower back pain. Her symptoms had started about three weeks previously, although she had been experiencing some problems ever since a serious car accident about 5 years before. She had also been suffering from intermittent pelvic pain for a few years, and severe pre-menstrual tension. On examination I found that there was an acute spasm of her lower back muscles, and that the mobility of some of her lumbar vertebrae was restricted. On palpation of her lower abdomen there was a lot of sensitivity and muscle guarding, particularly on the left side. When I tuned in to the tidal motion of fluid in the region, there was a strong sense of echoing which seemed to emanate from her left ovary. This fluid motion felt quite disorganized. I recommended that Rachel undergo some further tests to establish the cause of this finding. A couple of weeks later a pelvic scan revealed the presence of a benign tumour of the left ovary.

I suggested that we could try to work with this problem using craniosacral approaches, and Rachel agreed. We started the treatment by facilitating the expression of primary respiratory motion in the tissues of her lower back and pelvis. Her lower spine was very tight and there was a strong pull in the connective tissues of her pelvis, which was causing it to twist. It seemed that this was resulting in her left ovary getting compressed, restricting its ability to take up the Breath of Life. Some of these patterns felt easier after a few treatment sessions.

I then tried to re-establish the expression of potency in her left ovary. To do this I gently encouraged fluid and potency towards the ovary by facilitating a lateral fluctuation between my two hands, placed either side at the front and back (the encouragement of lateral fluctuations can be used for treatment as well as diagnosis). As I did this Rachel felt some pulsing in the left side of her pelvis, followed by a deep sense of relaxation and opening.

Two months later, Rachel went for further tests to investigate her condition and was told that the tumour had greatly reduced. She has continued to experience an improvement in her back problem, and also no longer suffers from the previously debilitating symptoms of pre-menstrual tension.

Fascial glide

Another skill commonly used for diagnosis is to engage the body's internal network of connective tissue, the fascia, in a 'conversation'. In health, the fascial tissues of the body are able to glide against each other, allowing mobility between all the different organs which they envelop. However, adhesions can form, reducing this capacity to glide. As fascia is relatively inelastic, resistances can easily be transmitted from one area of the body to another. This can be a significant cause of inertia affecting primary respiratory motion.

Due to the unbroken continuity of fascial tissue in the body, it is possible to palpate resistances to motion from one end of this network to the other. To do this the practitioner places his hands over, say, the patient's feet and senses into the underlying fascial tissues. A light suggestion of traction can then be introduced through the hands by subtly suggesting an inferior motion of the fascia (i.e. towards the patient's feet). The fascia's response is then assessed. If there is no resistance, fascia will easily be able to accommodate for this gentle suggestion of traction and the tissues will glide towards the feet accordingly. However, any inertia is felt as resistance to the fascia's natural gliding motion.

By holding any one part of the fascial network, the whole system is contacted, making it possible to locate the site of any resistance even in distant areas of the body. One old-timer, who had been practising cranial work for many years, was able to feel and accurately locate cranial restrictions, through the continuity of fascial tissue, in just the few seconds it took to shake your hand![40]

PERCEPTION

The real voyage of discovery consists not in seeking
new landscapes but in having new eyes.
MARCEL PROUST

Perceptual viewpoints

In the biodynamic approach of craniosacral work, there is an acknowledgement of different tidal expressions of the Breath of Life, i.e. the 'three tides'. Each of these unfoldments requires a different perceptual skill for both diagnosis and treatment. In the process of tuning in to a patient's system, what is actually perceived is determined by the 'glasses' that are being looked through. As with a radio, the practitioner can listen to different frequencies or unfoldments of a person's system by adjusting his 'tuning-in button'. For example, if the practitioner's perception is tuned in to how the cranial bones 'float like corks' on the tide, then he will probably notice their patterns of flexion and extension, etc. If he tunes in to the motility of tissues, he will perhaps notice their inner breathing. If he is able to drop his attention into the forces beneath these tissue patterns, he may notice the motion of one of the slower tides. What we 'see' is what we get. If a person's inherent health is tuned in to, it will surely be found. However, if we focus on problems and pathologies, that's what we'll see!

A story from China illustrates this principle. A wise old woman lived just outside a large town. Every day she would take her goats and sheep out to pasture in the nearby hills. While her animals grazed, she liked to sit on a rock overlooking the path to the town. One day when she was on this rock, a traveller came along the path. Looking up, he noticed the old woman and approached her. He asked if he was heading in the right direction for the town, and she replied that indeed he was. He then enquired, 'What are the people like in this town?' The old woman answered, 'What were people like in the town where you have just come from?' The traveller said, 'Oh! They were terrible! Everybody was fighting each other, there were awful jealousies and people were generally very unfriendly. That's why I'm thinking of moving to a new town.' The old woman replied, 'Well, I think you will find people are pretty much the same here, too.'

A few hours later another traveller passed along the path and he, too, looked up at the old woman to ask her for directions. He then asked, 'What are the people like in this town?' The old woman again replied, 'What were people like in the town where you have just come from?' 'Oh!', he said, 'They were wonderful! Everybody was very friendly and took great care of each other. You could really feel their warmth and generosity.' The old woman answered, 'Well, I think you will find people are pretty much the same here, too.'[41]

Observer and the observed

To some degree craniosacral work is always subjective, as it is based on what arises within the particular relationship formed between patient and practitioner. In all our human relationships we can see how different people bring out different qualities within us. In quantum physics it is well recognized that the observer of an experiment can affect its results. The experimenter is an inextricable part of the experiment, and cannot be separated from what is being observed. The observer's choices about how and what to measure will determine what is found.

To give a classic example, there are different experiments in physics which can investigate whether light is composed of particles or waves. However, some of these experiments inarguably prove that light is composed of particles, while others clearly show that it is composed of waves. Either can be proved, according to how light is observed. The nature of light can thus be described as either a wave or a particle, depending on the machine that is measuring it. Therefore, whether light is seen as a particle or a wave is totally dependent on the intention of the experimenter.[42]

Patient and the practitioner

If different practitioners operate with exactly the same diagnostic criteria, they will no doubt concur in their findings.[43] However, some individual variables are almost bound to enter, as both the practitioner and the patient are subjective parts of this process. This is why ten different practitioners can all put their hands on the same patient and perceive the patient's condition from a different perspective. Consequently, each one will probably get a different result from treatment, according to how the patient's system is met. None of these practitioners is necessarily wrong, but each one may be operating from a different 'perceptual field'.

Wide perceptual field

Imagine that you are standing at a bus stop, waiting for a bus. As you look down the road a question goes out, 'Is there a bus coming?' In the distance you see your bus approaching ... 'Yes, it's coming!' With a wide perceptual field, you ask a question and information comes back. How you hold your field of awareness will determine what you notice. However, let's say you are late for an interview and starting to get anxious; you may then miss the fact that it's a sunny day and the birds are singing. Alternatively, if you hold no focus because you're daydreaming, or if you are preoccupied with looking at the bus timetable, you may even miss the fact that the bus has arrived.[44] It is the same when a practitioner palpates a patient's primary respiratory system. For example, if he becomes focused only on bones, he may miss the longitudinal motion of fluid. Furthermore, if he makes a perceptual shift by widening his field of view, different information about the patient may become available.

Shifting perceptual fields

The practitioner can develop the ability to make intentional shifts in his perception in order to sense the different aspects of the primary respiratory system. This process of expanding or narrowing the field of perception can facilitate the ability to tune in to each of the three tides. With a relatively narrow perceptual field, the faster rhythmic rate of the cranial rhythmic impulse is more likely to be sensed. The slower tides of the Breath of Life are generally only palpable when the practitioner is operating with a wider field of perception. This involves an expansion of awareness, instead of focusing just on a particular part. When his perceptual field is widened to include the whole sense or 'whole biosphere' of the patient, the practitioner may be able to sense the slower mid-tide.[45] From this perspective it is easier to sense the underlying forces that organize the tissues.

It is then possible for the practitioner to keep widening his perceptual field to include the whole of the room he's in, or even the whole of the district. Widening the perceptual field even further – that is, right out to the horizons – enables easier access to the subtle rhythm of the long tide. This is also the domain of the mythic and the region of our 'imaginal' experience.[46] With a wide field of perception, the unknown can make itself known.

Larger context

In craniosacral diagnosis and treatment, even though a wide perceptual field may be used, it is still possible to place attention at a specific place or to notice a particular structure in the body. However, the context of this information becomes larger. Working with this sense of space is not the same as 'spacing out'. It is about remembering the universal while not losing sight of the particular. There is a wonderful old Sufi saying, 'Remember the Infinite, but don't forget to tie up your camel!' Essentially, this is an interplay between *attention* and *awareness*. Awareness is our sense of the whole, and attention is our recognition of the specific. Gabrielle Roth remarks, 'Ideally, attention should be a point of consciousness moving around inside the field of awareness. Awareness is the forest, attention is the trees.'[47]

A perceptual exercise

In a seated position, with your eyes either open or closed, establish your 'practitioner fulcrums' (see earlier section). Imagine a line continuing from the base of your spine down into the ground beneath you, like you are dropping an anchor into the earth. Then imagine another line going from the back of your head diagonally down into the ground behind you, at an angle of about 30 degrees. Let yourself settle with these fulcrums for a few moments.

Notice how you are breathing in and out, without trying to change anything. Place your attention into the sensations of your body. Do you breathe in more easily, or breathe out more easily? Are there particular sensations that you notice in your body as you breathe? These may be pleasant, or there may be places which feel uncomfortable – simply notice them.

Notice what takes you away from being aware of your breathing and your sensations. Maybe you start thinking about what you are going to eat for dinner, or about something you have to do, or you start noticing sounds in the room, or from outside. When you become aware that your attention has wandered, gently bring it back to your breathing and your sensations. See if the coming and going of your attention settles somewhere – that is, finds a point of balance, your 'practitioner neutral'.

Now widen your field of perception by allowing your awareness to take in the whole sense of yourself. What do you notice as you include your whole body and its field of energy in your awareness?

Gradually expand your awareness even further to include the whole of the room you are in. Pay attention to what you notice within this wider perceptual field. How does this change the sense you have of yourself?

Let the domain of your awareness spread out beyond the room, into the surrounding area and out towards the horizons. However, this does not mean that you have to leave your body – you are simply paying attention within a wider context. As you let your awareness expand towards the horizons, what do you notice?

Slowly bring your awareness back into the room by narrowing your perceptual field, and then bring it back into particular sensations in your body. Finally, take a little time to notice the rhythm of your breathing once more. We will now look at how this skill of shifting perceptual fields can be used in craniosacral work.

Perception of the mid-tide

The mid-tide is expressed as a rhythmic motion which can be palpated as a force within the fluids and tissues of the body. It is an expression of our biodynamic potency and has a stable rate of about 2.5 cycles per minute. This potency is initially taken up in the cerebrospinal fluid and produces its longitudinal fluctuation. It is the force which directly underlies the cranial rhythmic impulse. A patient who perceived the mid-tide during a treatment described the sensation as 'like being held in the palm of a hand and gently rocked by the life force'.[48] The mid-tide can most easily be perceived with a perceptual field that includes the whole physical and energetic make-up of the person.

A mid-tide exercise

Sit comfortably and place your hands lightly on the upper surface of your thighs. Begin by simply listening to any impressions which come into your hands. Then, start to feel any qualities in the tissues directly underlying your hands. Let your fingers rest on these 'corks floating on the tide' and see if you can sense the subtle motion of the cranial rhythmic impulse in your legs. You may need to narrow your field of attention into the tissues under your hands in order to feel their particular pattern of motion, but this should be done in a very relaxed way and with a soft focus.

Once you have a sense of how the tissues are expressing their craniosacral motion, start to tune in to the fluid under your hands. Imagine your hands are resting on the surface of a balloon filled with fluid, and see if you can palpate its fluctuating motion as the fluid moves longitudinally into inhalation and exhalation.

Then, widen your perceptual field to include a whole sense of yourself. Let your attention broaden out into awareness. Move your interest from an appreciation of just the outer motion of tissues and fluid, and start to sense the force or vitality expressed within. To do this, keep your mind relatively still and relaxed and imagine your hands are actually immersed in the fluid. In this way it is possible to place your awareness into the potency forces carried within the fluid. At this level of perception you may notice the rhythmic motion of the mid-tide operating at a slower rate. You may feel it as a subtle surge and settling of potency, fluid and tissues as they move into inhalation and exhalation.

Gently narrow your perceptual field again and notice how the cranial rhythmic impulse is being expressed by the tissues under your hands. When finishing this exercise, take time to re-orientate by taking a few deep breaths and having a gentle stretch before getting up.

Unified motion

Perhaps with a little practice, the mid-tide can be palpated as a field of motion which permeates the fluid and is organized around the midline of the body. Through the medium of the body's fluid, it produces an inner breathing or motility of tissues. At this level of function, tissues, fluid and potency all breathe together as 'one thing'.[49] This rhythmic expression of biodynamic potency organizes the function of cells and tissues, and carries our blueprint for health. Palpating the mid-tide gives the practitioner important clinical information about the essential forces which organize our health, and how they operate in relation to any stress or trauma.

When palpating the mid-tide, any inertia is perceived as a distortion within this unified field of motion, organized around an inertial fulcrum. Within every inertial fulcrum there is a concentration or gathering of trapped potency, consisting of the biodynamic and biokinetic forces which centre and maintain the disturbance. These are the forces which underlie any tissue contractions or compressions. It is the presence of these concentrations of trapped potency which affect the natural balance of the mid-tide.

At the level of the mid-tide, an inertial fulcrum may be perceived as a concentration or gathering of inertial potency, underlying a pattern of restricted motion in the tissues. However, if the same condition is tuned in to at the level of the cranial rhythmic impulse, it may be discerned as, say, a flexion pattern or an external rotation pattern, etc. A person tuning in to the mid-tide will not necessarily perceive which type of pattern a particular structure is holding, but will be aware of its general shape, and the forces which organize and underlie it.

Perception of the long tide

The long tide is the initial tidal unfoldment of the Breath of Life, emerging from intrinsic stillness. It has a very light and airy quality, as it rhythmically 'breathes' into inhalation and exhalation in 100-second cycles. This is the most subtle radiance of the Breath of Life, which expresses our original matrix of health. To access a perception of the long tide it is necessary to be very still and relaxed, and to hold a very wide field of perception. Dr James Jealous suggests that you let your awareness breathe right out towards the horizons.[50] When the long tide makes itself apparent, it is usually a sign of some deep settling and integration taking place in the patient's primary respiratory system. Consequently it cannot always be palpated. However, the exercise below may enable us to perceive this phenomenon.

A long tide exercise

Continuing from the last exercise, let your hands gently rest on your thighs. Now, let the horizons of your awareness expand around you, not only appreciating the whole sense of yourself but also taking in the whole room, the building, the street and the area you're in. Let this expansion happen gradually by allowing your perceptual field to breathe out naturally. Essentially, this is a process of letting go and cannot be achieved by effort.

From your perception of the mid-tide in the last exercise, imagine that your hands are immersed in the potency you may have sensed before. See if you can perceive the underlying force of the long tide, enfolded within the mid-tide.

To access the long tide it is necessary to be very still and relaxed, and to have a very light quality of awareness. Try to let go of looking for anything, but just let impressions come into your hands. The long tide has a very subtle quality of radiance as it gently permeates the tissues. You may feel it as a shimmering which comes into your hands, slowly moving into inhalation and exhalation in 100-second cycles. At this level of perception, inertia is perceived as slight distortions within the 'fabric' of this subtle field of motion.

Slowly narrow your perceptual field again, bringing your awareness back into the mid-tide, and then again to the cranial rhythmic impulse. Take a few moments to notice the sensations which you feel before slowly getting up.

Perception of dynamic stillness

If we are able to still ourselves even more deeply, we may be able to sense the dynamic stillness which is at the basis of all primary respiratory motion. Perception of this primordial state is an infrequent and precious event, but we may sometimes catch glimpses of it. First, however, we may have to clear some of our perceptual clutter! As Lao Tzu observed, 'In silence the teachings are heard.'

This state can be experienced as something within us which is universal, beyond the duality of subject or object. It has no defining characteristics or qualities, as it is the realm of our pure unfabricated nature. Consequently there are no words or concepts which can adequately describe it. At this level of our being there is no inertia and no conditioning, just the presence of peace, luminosity and stillness.

Tracking the changes

Craniosacral diagnosis involves following living and dynamic processes as they unfold within the patient. During the course of treatment it is important for the practitioner to note what changes are taking place as things proceed. For example, has there been a resolution of the forces trapped at the inertial fulcrum, or is the fulcrum still exerting an influence? Do the tissues express any greater ease of motility and mobility? Tracking the changes enables the practitioner to follow any resolution within a patient and to quantify what still remains to be worked with.

In principle, this process need not even end at death, for the Breath of Life never dies. Once it has left the body, the Breath of Life still continues to function. In the Tibetan Buddhist tradition the intermediate states between one life and the next are known as *bardo* states. There are many Tibetan *lamas* who are adept in the practice of tracking and supporting the departing life-stream during its journey through the bardo states after death.[51]

A *lifetime's practice*

The refinement of palpatory and perceptual skills is a lifetime's work (at least!); it requires a great deal of practice to cultivate. With practice, the ability to differentiate between many subtleties within the primary respiratory system can be achieved. This skill has the potential to reveal the presence of disease processes at their most profound level of physiological functioning. As Dr Magoun points out, X-rays may show gross changes in pathology, and laboratory tests can analyse changes in body chemistry, but neither can reveal the fine and subtle shades of motion, tone and tension in the tissues.[52]

Diagnosis becomes treatment

The dividing line between where diagnosis ends and treatment starts is not always well defined. As we noted, just the simple act of presence and contact can create change. A kindly hand on the shoulder may be enough to help someone work things out when distressed, and just the ability to identify a problem can be the start of its transformation. Once we perceive how we have become conditioned by a stressful experience, we have already begun to work with the issue. The practitioner's ability to clearly reflect this conditioning can act as an important resource in the process of our own healing and resolution. In this way diagnosis becomes treatment; one very naturally flows into the other.

7

ESSENTIALS OF
TREATMENT

To find health should be the object of the physician.

Anyone can find disease.[1]

DR A. T. STILL

AIMS OF TREATMENT

A doctor who prescribes an identical treatment in two
individuals and expects an identical development, may
be properly classified as a social menace.
LIN YUTANG

'It seemed like he was hardly doing anything' ... 'I just lay there as he put his hands on my head, but when I got up it felt like there was more wind in my sails' ... 'I don't know what was going on, but my back pain disappeared afterwards.' These are all comments heard from patients after receiving craniosacral treatment. It can be a surprise, if not a culture shock, to realize that inside of us we have all the resources that are needed for healing. We are so used to asking doctors to 'do something' to make us feel better that we often lose sight of our own inner potential.

From the outside, at least, nothing much seems to be going on during a craniosacral treatment. For many minutes at a time, the practitioner's hands may rest in gentle contact with the patient's body. Yet as a result of the application of subtle skills, a great deal can happen at a profound level of physiological functioning. As Hugh Milne remarks, 'It's amazing how much how little will do.'[2]

There are many different treatment approaches employed in craniosacral work, but they all have one thing in common. *They all work with the essential forces of health found within the patient.* The practitioner's attention is placed on the rhythmic motions of the Breath of Life and how they are able to bring order into the body. The main intention of treatment is to find, support and facilitate these expressions of health. When the Breath of Life finds expression in areas of disorder, motion resumes and health is restored. In this process discordant parts of ourselves, which have become separated from their source of order and vitality, are brought back into relationship with the whole. We literally become more of who we are.[3]

Supporting health

Health is at the foundation of our being. Although the essential forces of health are never actually lost, they have to re-organize in relationship to the experiences in life which shape us – mental, emotional and physical. Sometimes an experience (such as an accident, trauma or toxin) overwhelms our ability to dissipate its effects, and inertia is the result. Health then organizes itself, seeking the best possible balance in the circumstances. But there is still health; there is still life. To work with our health means not limiting our attention to what is wrong, but identifying with and supporting what works. Finding the health in the patient gives the practitioner some deep-acting and tangible resources to work with.

In craniosacral treatment, the patient's intrinsic forces of health are relied upon to make any necessary change, rather than the practitioner applying some external force.[4] In this regard, Dr John Upledger observes, 'I realize that my job is as a facilitator to the patient's own healing process.'[5] Nevertheless, the skill of the practitioner is an important element within this healing process. It seems that, without some help, our healing resources cannot always be accessed. The clear reflection and support provided by a practitioner's hands may be the particular key which unlocks the door to health.

Meeting the needs

Craniosacral work is a client-centred approach, as treatment is tailored to individual needs. Listening and responding to the messages given by the physiology of the patient enables the practitioner to relate to conditions with appropriateness and safety. It is always therefore the patient's own physiology which dictates how and where treatment is applied. In this way, treatment is simply followed in a fluid process rather than prescribed or predicted.

Prescriptive approaches based on protocols of treatment and the application of techniques are never as effective as following the priorities of the Breath of Life itself. The way that an inertial pattern can be unlocked is individual and unique, and needs to suit the particular conditions of the patient at that time. The Tibetans seem to understand this principle well, for the word for 'health' in traditional Tibetan medicine is *trowaten*, which literally translates as 'that which suits you'.

STATES OF BALANCE

*When the human mind-emotion-body continuum comes into alignment
with life's intrinsic order, there is an avenue for the release of an
immensity of power.*[6]
MICHAEL BURGHLEY

Patterns and fulcrums

Each pattern of stress in the body is organized around an inertial fulcrum which acts as its centre of disturbance. At the core of each inertial fulcrum there is a concentration of trapped potency. Due to these bound-up forces, patterns of compression, twists and pulls become retained in the tissues. Wherever inertial forces are concentrated, the expression of the essential ordering principle of the Breath of Life is affected. As a result, a lot of energy which would otherwise be available to the whole system can get bound up. It is the aim of any treatment to help free this up.

To be effective, treatment has to deal with the origin of a problem, its fulcrum, not just the symptoms or effects. In order to resolve a tissue contraction there must be a resolution of the underlying forces trapped at its fulcrum. Unless these forces are dissipated, the pattern will continue in some shape or form. Therefore, by noticing changes which take place at the inertial fulcrum the practitioner is able to track any real progress. It should be noted that tissues can sometimes change their pattern of motion, without any significant change occurring at the fulcrum itself. However, one of the tenets of craniosacral practice is that all true healing occurs at the fulcrum organizing the disturbance.

Point of balanced tension

The *point of balanced tension* describes the optimal alignment in the tissues for an inertial fulcrum to resolve. It is a particular point which can be found within the range of motion of a tissue pattern. In effect, it is the position at which there is a balance between the natural forces expressed in the tissues and any increased tensions added as a result of a stress or strain. Remember that the biodynamic potency of the Breath of Life is the intrinsic natural force within the body. In addition, the body contains the forces of any added stresses it has retained – the biokinetic potencies. The point of balanced tension is a position of the tissues at which all these forces gathered around a fulcrum become balanced. This is the point at which a stress pattern is maintaining its focus.

Imagine a circular see-saw with children sitting all around it. The point of balanced tension is where the weight of all the children is evenly distributed around the central fulcrum point.[7] In the body, it is at this point that there is the least possible resistance in the tissues and the minimal amount of 'push and pull'. Dr Magoun describes it as, 'The most neutral position possible under the influence of all the factors responsible for the existing pattern.'[8] It can also be compared to putting the gears of a car in neutral.[9] When this point is reached, the tissues settle into stillness.

When a point of balanced tension is found, the self-healing and self-regulating forces of the body can most easily come back into play. Once there is no force or tension being exerted in one direction or another, the forces held within an inertial fulcrum have an opportunity to resolve. Therefore, by accessing this point a doorway is created through which a re-organization of an inertial pattern can take place.

The point of balanced tension can be accessed within a tissue's normal range of motion. Therefore, there are no added forces that need to be introduced from the outside. This neutral position is unique for each strain pattern in the body[10] and, given the opportunity, the tissues naturally seek to move towards this point. However, they may be rendered unable to do so by forces in the body that have become inertial. It is then that the gentle hands-on encouragement of a practitioner may be required.

Accessing the stillness

When the point of balanced tension is reached, a stillness occurs as the tissues settle into their neutral position. This is sometimes called a *local stillpoint*. The stillness is a gateway through which our potential for healing can be found. It is within this stillness that the body can access and express its intrinsic resources of health. This is the key to unlocking inertial forces trapped in the body.

Accessing the stillness at a point of balanced tension is the first objective that the practitioner seeks during treatment. One of the main ways to encourage this point is to suggest a slowing down in the patterns of craniosacral motion. This is done by the introduction of subtle suggestions or invitations into the tissues from the practitioner's hands.

As the tissues move towards a point of balanced tension, pulsations, vibrations or other motions sometimes appear as a re-organization starts to take place. When the trapped potency is released, heat is often given off. It is also at this point that old memories locked in the tissues can come to the surface and begin their process of resolution. Therefore, stressful experiences which the body may have been unable to integrate previously may be revisited at another point. If the body is then able to access the necessary resources, the dissipation of trapped potencies and the process of healing can be completed.

The point of balanced tension is essentially a position at which the body can make its own adjustments. When it is reached, the practitioner need only wait for the intrinsic forces of the patient's own physiology to get to work. This is marked by the mobilization of potency trapped at the fulcrum and a restoration of primary respiratory motion.

Inherent treatment plan

As we noted, tissues involved in an inertial pattern have a natural tendency to seek a point of balanced tension. This tendency is the result of our intrinsic biodynamic forces, which always seek optimal health no matter what the conditions. If the practitioner can identify how the body naturally attempts to seek balance and resolve its inertia, this process can simply be supported in the form of a gentle facilitation introduced through the hands. However, the practitioner need only follow the process being led by their patient's own physiology, as their tissues, fluids and potencies move towards a resolution. These natural priorities manifest within the patterns of primary respiratory motion, and are referred to as the *inherent treatment plan*.

It sometimes takes many minutes of 'listening' and palpation with a wide perceptual field before the inherent treatment plan is revealed. The inertial fulcrums that significantly influence primary respiratory motion then become displayed as major focal points at which there is a gathering of forces. This is because the organizing biodynamic forces in the body start to work with inertial fulcrums in an order of priority. It may seem uncanny, but the natural wisdom in the body unfailingly knows what it needs next to find optimal balance.

In this approach, the patient is looked at from the inside-out, rather than from the outside-in.[11] As an outsider looking in, it's usually more difficult to know what needs to happen, but as an insider looking out it's easier to follow the natural priorities of treatment as they unfold. On following this principle, Dr Jealous states,

> *We use our hands diagnostically, perceptually, and therapeutically – that's*
> *how simple and profound this is. We are not listening for symptoms but for*
> *a pre-established priority set in motion by the Health of the patient.*[12]

The inherent treatment plan is, actually, the easiest possible way that a particular pattern can resolve.[13] Therefore, following this priority has practical and effective clinical consequences. One ramification is that the place where treatment is most effectively given is not necessarily where the patient is currently experiencing their symptoms.[14] To give an illustration, let's say that a patient has lower back pain. The practitioner may make contact at the lower back to tune in to what is happening there, but as he widens his perceptual field he may become aware of patterns in other areas of the body.

For example, the practitioner may notice a gathering of inertial forces in the diaphragm and a contraction of tissues in that area. After a point of balanced tension is facilitated in this pattern, some tissue activity may then start up in the neck. Placing attention there, some fast tremors may occur, indicative of held-in shock dissipating from the tissues, perhaps from an old injury. When that has ceased, the whole upper spine may re-organize and readjust towards a better alignment with the midline. Finally, and perhaps only then, something may start to resolve at the lower back. The point is that the practitioner could not have known in advance the order in which these things needed to resolve. The treatment plan was only revealed by following the priorities and intelligence of the patient's own primary respiratory system.[15]

Following the inherent treatment plan is a great support to the patient's intrinsic and intelligent forces of health. However, in order to do this, both patient and practitioner may have to let go of their concepts and projections about what they think *should* happen. Only then can this deeper intelligence be appreciated. The Breath of Life itself provides the design for health. The superb intelligence of this design can be followed by simply being open to the way in which these forces wish to move. Dr Becker explains,

> We have ... to allow physiological function within the patient to literally train us. We seek to learn: Where is the health in this patient? How do I get it to the surface? The body physiology is literally training us.[16]

Trusting the wisdom

Working with the inherent and natural forces of the body, is not only the most real and effective way of supporting cure, but also prevents harm from occurring. It works with what Dr Becker called 'the bioenergy of wellness ... the most powerful force in the world'.[17] This intrinsic force in the body can always be relied upon to give the most appropriate help needed. Nevertheless, learning to trust this wisdom can at times be challenging.

I was treating a woman in her mid-forties during her first craniosacral therapy appointment. She had come with a pain in her mid-back and right shoulder blade, produced one month before while making a sudden turn when dancing. At the start of the session, I told her that I was going to tune in to the subtle motion of her body, initially with my hands gently cupping her head. As I moved into position, I sensed a tension. The back of her cranium felt tight and compressed, and after a couple of minutes she started to get agitated. I asked her how she was doing, but no answer came back.

After another minute I asked again, but still there was no reply. So I patiently waited with my hands on her head, giving her system a lot of space and tracking the sense of tension that I could feel. I started to notice the longitudinal fluctuation of her cerebrospinal fluid, which had a strong quality of fluid drive. This told me that her basic resources of health were good. Furthermore, I sensed that the major fulcrum which was organizing her tension pattern was at the floor of her cranium. It seemed that there was a gathering of inertial forces in this area, and the tissues in the upper part of her body were getting pulled towards this place. Her physiology was showing me that this was the source of her problem. After another minute or two, I asked again, 'How are you doing?'

No sooner had the words left my mouth than she forcefully snapped, 'You don't really want to know, do you?!' I replied, 'Yes I do ... that's why I'm asking!' Again there was silence. After another minute I rechecked how she was feeling. She then responded, 'Are you sure you want to know?!' Again I tried to give her reassurance. She angrily exclaimed, 'Well, I'm wondering what the hell you are doing with your hands on my head, when I've come to you with a pain in my back!!' Acknowledging the strength of her feeling, I said something like, 'Thank you for telling me. I can really sense your frustration around that!' She retorted, 'Yes! I'm really frustrated and angry!'

I thought to myself, either I trust what her body is showing me, or I just quit while I can and end the session here and now. Anyway, I decided to trust and continued the dialogue. I told her that I felt there was some tension at the base of her head which was probably influencing what she was feeling in her back, and asked her if she wanted to continue. She gave a little nod. I then suggested that she place her attention into the sensations of her body to see if there was a location where her feeling of frustration was getting held. After a short while she curtly declared, 'My back hurts and my head is tight.'

'How do you feel about staying in touch with those sensations right now?' I asked. Again, she gave a little nod. Within a few minutes some strong pulsations and twitches started to manifest in her head. I encouraged her to let these movements happen, while still supporting her head in my hands. At this point, she began to experience some painful feelings of neglect and started to cry. These were familiar emotions that she had encountered from time to time ever since she was a young girl. After some minutes she gradually settled, and the bones at the base of her skull reached a point of balanced tension. I could then feel her head literally coming back to life, as primary respiratory motion started to permeate the tissues. Soon after, she entered a state of deep relaxation and the whole region felt more open.

I again asked her how she was doing. 'Pretty good', came the reply, 'but I still feel some tension in my back.' I moved my hands to the area of complaint and started working with the local pattern affecting her spine and shoulder blade. With gentle facilitation, these tissues moved a little further into their contraction, gave a little twitch and then softened. She left the session 90 per cent symptom-free, and recovered fully within another couple of treatments.

Kernel of health

In the biodynamic approach of craniosacral work there is an appreciation of the forces which centre and maintain a problem. If these inertial forces can be dissipated, the whole pattern of disease which has become organized around the fulcrum changes. An appreciation of this level of physiological functioning goes right back to the very roots of osteopathy. Nearly a century ago, Dr Andrew Taylor Still remarked that essentially the role of the practitioner is to revive 'suspended forces', in the same way that an electrician works with electrical currents.[18]

When any of the natural forces in the body become inertial, they produce a disturbance of function. However, once these forces are mobilized they provide a deep resource for healing and transformation. Therefore, the inertial forces which centre a disturbance can be regarded as a *kernel of health* trapped within every fulcrum. This kernel of health is simply something which has to be liberated for healing to result. When forces are transformed from a state of inertia, a more wholesome connection of that region to the universal principle of the Breath of Life is established. The individual and separately functioning 'wave' realizes that it is part of the 'ocean' and re-enters the life-stream.

Eye of the needle

The point of balanced tension has been compared to 'the eye of the needle'.[21] It is an opening or gateway through which suspended forces are able to pass, in a similar way to how thread is passed through the eye of a needle. The threading of these suspended forces can be a palpable experience. As the Breath of Life permeates the tissues, it may be felt as just a trickle at first, then perhaps a bubbling, followed by a stream, until the tissues breathe openly and primary respiratory motion is restored. During this process one young boy described how he could feel his face literally changing shape as his birth trauma started to resolve. 'It's just like in the film *The Mask*!', he exclaimed.[22]

The stillness at the point of balanced tension is a doorway which can open up to even deeper levels of primary respiratory function. It can be seen as a kind of 'pregnant pause' full of healing potential and from which new life can emerge. Perceptions of deeper tidal forces and of more profound states of stillness can unfold from this place. Thus, the eye of the needle is like a gateway to other realms of experience, a 'crack between the worlds'.[23] Through this gateway, deeper states of being can become apparent.

States of balance

As we pass through the eye of the needle provided by the point of balanced tension, a set-tling and reconnection with our deeper forces of health can occur. At this point, it is common to experience the slower rhythms of the mid-tide and the long tide, which can then come more into relationship with our everyday physiological functioning. This process of passing through the gateway into deeper levels of function is referred to by Franklyn Sills as accessing *'states of balanced tension'*.[24] In states of balanced tension, a transformation of inertial patterns can occur as we become touched by deeper aspects of the Breath of Life and its inherent healing principle.

At a *point* of balanced tension, tissues find a neutral place of stillness, but in *states* of bal-anced tension a neutral is found in the deeper forces that organize these tissue patterns. Points of balanced tension occur at the level of the cranial rhythmic impulse, but states of balanced tension refer to a neutral state which can be accessed within the deeper unfold-ments of the Breath of Life. This may be a progressive process, as balance is found first in the cranial rhythmic impulse, then the mid-tide and then the long tide, perhaps eventually lead-ing to a reconnection with the dynamic stillness at the basis of all function. The settling into deeper and deeper states of balance leads us to the very heart of healing.[25]

Three-step healing process

With the benefit of many years of clinical experience, Dr Rollin Becker recognized that the process of treatment can be simply broken down into three essential phases.[19] The first phase involves a recognition that the tissues, fluids and biodynamic potencies of the patient naturally seek states of balanced tension. There is an inherent tendency towards this balance which the practitioner either simply needs to follow, or perhaps gently support by providing some facilitation.

Phase two is when a state of balanced tension is reached, which Dr Becker calls a 'pause-rest period'.[20] It is marked by a temporary stilling of tissue motion. This stillness is the essence of the therapeutic process. It is the optimal state in which inertial forces can be resolved. When tissue motion restarts from this state of stillness, something changes.

The third, and last, phase of treatment is when primary respiratory motion resumes within the tissues after a change has taken place. When this happens there is a shift towards a better balance and symmetry of motion around its natural fulcrums. The practitioner can then track the changes that have taken place and assess any inertia remaining.

Here's a summary of the three-step healing process:

Phase One   Tissues, fluids and potencies seek a state of balanced tension.
Phase Two   A state of balance is reached and 'something happens'.
Phase Three   Motion resumes and a change takes place.

Summary of treatment skills

During treatment, the practitioner essentially follows and facilitates the intrinsic wisdom of the body as it seeks to resolve patterns of inertia. Accessing points or states of balanced tension in patterns of disorder is at the core of this healing process. In this regard, the following skills need to be developed:

- the ability to perceive the expressions of primary respiratory motion which maintain physiological function and health
- the ability to sense inertial patterns which affect primary respiratory motion
- the ability to sense the location of inertial fulcrums which organize these patterns
- the ability to help the patient access points and states of balanced tension
- the ability to perceive the mobilization of suspended forces contained within the inertial fulcrum
- the ability to assess changes that take place.

THERAPEUTIC SKILLS

If you understand the mechanism, your technique is simple.[26]
DR W. G. SUTHERLAND D.O.

Although the primary respiratory system functions as an integrated whole, particular skills are required to relate to its different aspects. Varying degrees of facilitation, as well as diverse skills of perception, are needed according to which of the three tides is being worked with. For example, when working at the level of the mid-tide or the long tide, *less active* skills of treatment are generally sufficient. When relating to these deeper unfoldments of the Breath of Life it is easier for the practitioner simply to be a follower of the inherent treatment plan. This is because at these levels of physiological functioning, the ordering forces of the Breath of Life are more apparent. However, when working with the faster cranial rhythmic impulse (C.R.I.), relatively more active skills of engagement may be needed.

Working with the C.R.I.

In Chapter 6 we looked at the different perceptual skills required to palpate each of the three tides. The practitioner may have different insights into the patient's condition, according to the perceptual field being worked with. A relatively narrow perceptual field is more likely to reveal the functioning of the C.R.I. Here, the practitioner may notice how individual structures of the body express their craniosacral motion, and how inertial forces create sites of restriction to this motion. For example, the particular way that the occiput expresses its flexion and extension can be assessed. At the C.R.I. level of physiological functioning, inertia of the occiput is perceived as a specific resistance (such as a compression or a pull) to the natural pattern of its craniosacral motion.

When working at the level of the C.R.I., a particular bone or membrane may need gentle yet relatively active suggestions transmitted to it via the practitioner's hands in order to access a point of balanced tension. Furthermore, other skills may be needed to relate to disturbances affecting the fluid systems of the body. When healing occurs, it is perceived as a freeing up of tissue resistances and restoration of craniosacral motion around its natural fulcrums. This is marked by a return of flexion/extension and external/internal rotation with more balance and symmetry. Some of the particular therapeutic skills which are employed to achieve these results will be explored in the next section (see Particular 'Conversations', page 166).

Mid-tide skills

The inertial potency which controls a pattern of disturbance is more easily appreciated when working with a relatively wide perceptual field in relationship to the mid-tide. At this level of perception, it's possible to go underneath the pattern of the forms to appreciate the forces that determine their function.[27] When working with the mid-tide, less active skills of treatment are generally required to help the primary respiratory system access states of balance. At this level of physiology there is a unity in the functioning of tissues, bones, fluid and potency. This is because the mid-tide operates as a unified, tensile field of biodynamic potency expressed within the fluids found in all living tissues.

When working with the mid-tide, inertial fulcrums are not necessarily perceived as specific resistances between tissues (as with the cranial rhythmic impulse), but as condensations of potency and distortions within this tensile field of activity. These distortions can affect the mid-tide's natural orientation around the midline of the body.

Here, the emphasis of treatment usually involves simply following the natural unfoldment of the inherent treatment plan, as the ordering forces of the body get to work. In addition, the practitioner can offer subtle suggestions of settling and space with his hands to facilitate states of balance. These suggestions are directed towards the slower motion patterns within tissues and fluids to help them find their neutral. In this way, the biodynamic forces expressed within the mid-tide, and those biokinetic forces influencing it, can reach a state of balance. When this occurs the mid-tide has an opportunity to realign towards the midline, and the expression of the Breath of Life can be restored. As a result of the resolution of these underlying forces, which have become inertial, tissue contractions release, nerve function becomes normalized, circulation improves ... and pathologies resolve. Shift happens!

Long tide skills

In the long tide, inertial patterns are perceived as subtle distortions within the matrix of this deepest expression of the Breath of Life. When the practitioner works with a wide perceptual field and a quality of deep stillness, an opportunity may be created for the long tide to show itself. When treating at this level of functioning, the practitioner can simply *be* with the patient's system and watch the changes unfold. Once the long tide emerges there is nothing for the practitioner to do, other than humbly witness these subtlest forces of primary respiratory motion. *Resonance* is the key therapeutic principle here. Healing may be perceived as a transformation of inertia from within, as the tissues become infused with the deeper resources of the Breath of Life. Dr Becker described this process in the following way:

> It took a full minute and a half for this larger tide to come in and be part of the body physiology of the patient, and then it drained away just as slowly as it came in. Where it came from and where it went, I do not know, but its influence was certainly modifying the trophism [i.e. nourishment] of every cell of the body to do something. For that patient, that trophism was certainly a help because the clinical response was that of an improvement in the areas of dysfunction.[28]

Dynamic stillness

Dynamic stillness is at the foundation of all the tidal motions of the Breath of Life. This is the realm from which all motion and expressions of life emerge. At this level of being there is no duality. There is no separation between tissues, fluids and potency, or between the practitioner and patient. Therefore, there is no 'treatment'. This is ground zero. Healing can occur instantaneously as patterns of experience become touched by this deepest level of being. This is an enigmatic and powerful event. It may be felt as a sense of grace, marked by the kind of silence that can be cut with a knife.[29]

A glimpse of stillness

In Asia, there is a tradition for students to learn how to directly experience their own intrinsic stillness under the guidance of a spiritual teacher. An old teaching story illustrates how it may be possible to come to know this indescribable realm.[30]

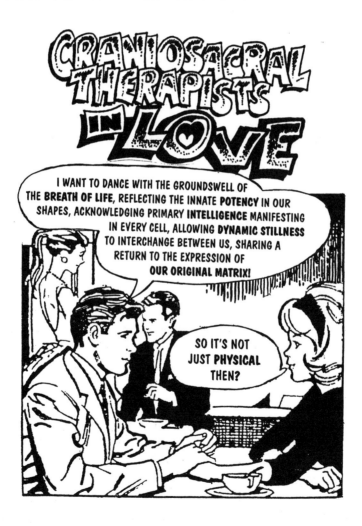

Figure 7.1: Craniosacral Therapists in Love (cartoon by Biff; text by Michael Kern)

There was a student who was very bright, but perhaps a little over-zealous. At every opportunity he asked his teacher to explain the nature of 'dynamic stillness'. Sometimes his teacher gave him a brief explanation, but often he just smiled and told the student to go and practise some more meditation. However, at their next meeting the student again asked, 'What is the nature of dynamic stillness?' Once more the teacher told him to practise more meditation.

One day, as his teacher was preparing for a large ceremony, the student again asked, 'What is the nature of dynamic stillness?' By now the teacher was starting to get a little impatient with this persistent questioning. He enquired, 'Do you recognize the thought that you just had?' The student hesitated for a moment and replied, 'Yes, I do.' The teacher continued, 'Can you imagine that there is another thought that you are just about to have?' The student nodded. The teacher then asked, 'Can you imagine that there is a space between these two thoughts?' 'Yes!' replied the student.

'Well ... lengthen it!' said the teacher.

PARTICULAR 'CONVERSATIONS'

The data of techniques are fascinating, but not for the sake of themselves.
They are important only insofar as they enable us to dive into the well of
being, only insofar as they create access to being alive, only insofar as they
support and forward our being home, our journey to ourselves.[31]
DIANNE M. CONNELLY

Tissues holding inertia can be invited or gently coaxed into expressing their potentials of motion by gentle suggestions made through the practitioner's hands. For example, suggestions of settling and stillness, or reminders of forgotten options of movement may be introduced. These suggestions are like *conversations* between the practitioner's hands and the patient's body. They are a way of engaging tissues and fluids in a dialogue about their needs and priorities.

When such suggestions are made, the responses of the body are always listened for and respected. Treatment given in this way involves a fluid and dynamic communication between the patient's physiology and the practitioner, and the application of therapeutic skills rather than techniques. Dr Becker explains, 'Doing something to a problem is technique; working with an inherent mechanism within the problem is an application of a principle, not a technique.'[32] 'Conversation' skills are used to support the expression of intrinsic health found at the heart of every inertial fulcrum. When working at the level of the cranial rhythmic impulse, these skills may be relatively actively applied. When in relationship to the deeper tides, more subtle suggestions are usually offered.

Different 'conversations' can be used to treat different conditions and different parts of the primary respiratory mechanism. Two principal methods are employed: one is an *indirect* approach and the other a *direct* approach. The difference between these two approaches is in the direction of motion that is suggested into the tissues. However, both attempt to facilitate points or states of balanced tension, where the tensions around a fulcrum are at a minimum. We will now explore these basic approaches and some of their variations.

Indirect approaches

With an indirect approach of treatment, tissues are followed into their 'direction of preference'. This is the pathway along which a tissue or bone can most easily express its primary respiratory motion, despite the presence of inertia. In effect, this is in the direction of the strain pattern. It is also the path of least resistance. For example, if a bone is stuck in internal rotation, it is followed there (see Figure 7.2).

Dr Upledger describes this as an 'unlatching' principle. It is like opening a tight door latch, where it may first be necessary to follow the closure.[33] Another way to think about an indirect approach is to imagine a kite which has been caught up in the branches of a tree. If you try to free the kite by pulling on its string, you may entangle it even more in the branches. However, if you let off the slack by loosening the string, the wind may then blow the kite out of the tree. This rationale of treatment can help reduce resistances held in tissues, creating an opportunity to free the suspended forces trapped within an inertial fulcrum.

When tissues are followed into their direction of preference, the pattern which they are holding is essentially being reflected back. In this way, the practitioner acts as a kind of reflective mirror for the patient and their potential for change.[34] This is an important therapeutic

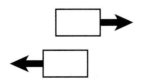

Figure 7.2: Indirect approach

principle, as much of the time we walk around unaware of our inertial patterns. It is often only when a pattern is reflected back that it is recognized and can become clarified. Franklyn Sills explains, 'In this reflection, something can be rediscovered that was forgotten, something can be reclaimed that was seemingly lost.'[35] This process is like shining a 'light' on the pattern, helping to bring it back into focus with the intrinsic biodynamic forces of the body.

There is always a natural boundary to how far a strain pattern can move. This is the point at which no more motion is possible without any extra force being added. It is marked by a subtle resistance to any further motion. When following a strain pattern, the practitioner always needs to recognize this boundary and take care not to press against it. However, it is at a place near the boundary that a point or state of balanced tension can often be found. It is here that the practitioner can most effectively introduce subtle suggestions into the tissues for them to settle into their neutral.

Exaggeration is another type of indirect approach, where the practitioner not only follows a tissue pattern into its direction of preference, but also gently amplifies this motion in a step-by-step process. Exaggeration can provide a stimulus for craniosacral motion and may help to increase its amplitude. This approach was the one used by Dr Sutherland to revive a drowning man by the shores of Lake Erie (see Chapter 1).[36] It may also trigger a kind of recoil in the tissues, helping them to spring back and self-correct. However, it is not used in many acute conditions such as recent trauma or headache, or where the symptoms might be aggravated by the exaggeration of the inertial pattern.[37]

Direct approaches

In this approach, points or states of balanced tension are sought by encouraging tissues to move directly *out* of their inertial pattern. Direct approaches help to remind tissues of their lost options. If tissues are stuck in one direction, motion is facilitated in the opposite direction. This can help counter any distortion and create space for the disengagement of an inertial pattern. For example, if a bone is stuck in internal rotation, a suggestion of external rotation is offered (see Figure 7.3). Suggestions of *traction* and *decompression* made into compressed tissues are also types of a direct approach.

When given the space, the self-corrective forces of the body have an opportunity to come back into play.[38] This is another important rationale of treatment. The common saying, 'time is a great healer' reflects this idea. In essence, time is equivalent to space. This understanding is well known in Ayurvedic medicine. According to the teachings of the 'Medicine Buddha' in an ancient Buddhist text, space is the most important and ultimate healing principle. This

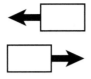

Figure 7.3: Direct approach

is because spaciousness is a fundamental quality of our natural state.[39] Therefore, creating space enables us to contact the source of our healing potential.

As tissues are gently facilitated to move out of their inertial pattern, their natural boundary of motion is respected. At or near this boundary, a settling and stillness can be encouraged by the practitioner's hands to help access a point/state of balanced tension, and provide an opportunity for re-organization. A student remarked that this was 'like having my forehead flossed'. One patient exclaimed, 'It feels like yoga from the inside!'[40]

Taking gravity off

Another common therapeutic approach is for the practitioner to lift and support a part of the body being treated to remove the effects of gravity. This is a particular type of indirect approach often used when working with the more freely movable regions of the body. For example, a limb can be supported by the practitioner, who tunes in to its pattern of primary respiratory motion. When the influence of gravity is removed, any strain patterns that tissues are holding may become more easily clarified. These patterns can then be followed into their direction of preference, and the tissues encouraged to access a point/state of balanced tension. The body as a whole can also be supported like this, although it usually requires the help of more than one practitioner to take the patient's weight.

Viola Frymann describes this process as similar to unravelling knots in a telephone flex: '... While the receiver remains on the instrument the distortion cannot change; an effort to pull it straight by direct action will be utterly useless ... The very simple measure, however, of taking the receiver off the instrument and permitting it to hang ... will enable the normalizing forces within to unwind that cord.'[41]

The motions which ensue when gravity is taken off are dictated by the particular tension patterns that the tissues are holding. Therefore, during this process the tissues are essentially

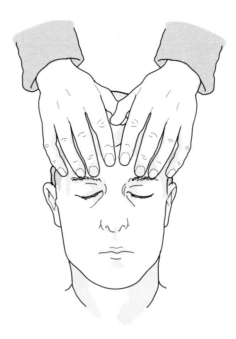

Figure 7.4: Hand contacts for working with the frontal bone

given an opportunity to express their pattern of trauma. The body will often move towards the position that it was in at the time of receiving the trauma. It is when in this position that a point/state of balanced tension may be found. For example, a patient who had slipped over on ice and broken his arm recreated this position while we followed the resultant inertial pattern into its direction of preference. It was only when his arm was in a twisted position, as it had been at the time he fell, that the inertial forces at the site of injury started to become mobilized. A re-organization then took place, relieving months of stiffness and pain.

'Unwinding'

This method was given the name *unwinding* by Dr Viola Frymann;[42] some craniosacral practitioners use it as a cardinal approach of treatment. Many people feel drawn to unwinding processes with the intention of reliving trauma patterns and completing any 'unfinished business'. When trauma patterns are followed, old memories and emotions associated with the experience held in the tissues often come to the surface. This frequently leads to cathartic responses as the patient attempts to discharge the trauma.

However, as a note of caution, when tissue patterns go into an unwinding process it doesn't necessarily mean that there is any resolution at their organizing fulcrum. Without a change occurring at the fulcrum, nothing significant has actually happened to change the pattern. This is like moving the furniture around in a room but still being stuck in the same living space. Furthermore, the re-experiencing of a trauma pattern may be too much for someone whose available healing resources are low. Therefore, the outcome may be retraumatization rather than benefit. We will look further at some of the ramifications of this approach in Chapter 9.

Intraosseous skills

Particular kinds of strain patterns may be retained within bony tissue, especially if a bone receives a trauma before it has fully ossified (see Chapter 10, A baby's skull, page 248). This type of pattern is called an *intraosseous lesion*. As a result, the bone's motility, or inner breathing, is affected.

Only direct approaches of treatment are used when working with intraosseous lesions. This is because these kinds of trauma patterns usually stem from an early age, before bones have fused and before any sutures have formed between them. Consequently, any boundaries to the practitioner's suggestion of motion are often unclear due to a lack of resistance (which the sutures would normally provide). As a result, there is a tendency for there to be no clear physiological boundary if an intraosseous pattern is followed into its direction of preference (i.e. using an indirect approach). The patient may then be just encouraged into their trauma pattern, rather than helped out of it. Furthermore, especially in the adult, the forces which maintain intraosseous lesions are often deeply entrenched, and so may require the facilitation of some space and disengagement.[43]

Light contact

The amount of pressure applied by the practitioner's hands is minimal. The tissues are invited, reminded or facilitated into finding a point/state of balanced tension in a spirit of enquiry, rather than with any coercion. Nothing is ever forced in craniosacral work. Dr Magoun confirms the need for subtlety and sensitivity: 'To employ other than skilful and delicate sense perception is to lose the shades of physiological reaction so necessary for success.'[44] He further describes,

One is reminded of the old fable of the North Wind and the Sun
attempting to remove the man's overcoat. The blustering gale only made
him wrap it more tightly about his body but the gentle warmth of the sun
soon effected the desired result.[45]

Imagine that you are standing on a tow path, trying to pull a barge through a canal lock with a rope. If you apply a sudden force on the rope, the barge will probably hardly move at all. It's more likely that the rope will either break, or you will rebound from the resistance provided by the barge and end up in the canal yourself! However, if you just lean forwards while holding the rope, this gentle and steady pressure will enable the barge to move slowly ahead. As Dr John Upledger observes, 'A small force over a long time can do more than a strong force over a short time. This is because the small force recruits much less resistance from the patient's body.'[46]

Although the vast majority of craniosacral treatment is carried out with an extremely light touch, on occasions stronger contacts may be appropriate. These occasions may include when resuscitating a patient, or working with the impact of physical trauma in the body.[47] A patient suffering from physical trauma may sometimes require a firmer contact to meet the strong forces locked in the body. However, the practitioner still does not apply any added force into the body, but only matches the forces already there. In this way, treatment is responsive rather than dictatorial.

Domino effect

In the biological sciences it has been proposed that all organisms live on an 'edge of chaos' and are therefore not very stable in their function. According to *Chaos Theory* it is thought that, for example, under certain conditions a butterfly flapping its wings on one side of the world could cause changes in the weather in the other! It seems that 'living systems are non-linear: in other words a small change in input to a living system can result in a large change in outcome.'[48] This has become known as the butterfly effect in Chaos Theory. In craniosacral work, a gentle encouragement in the right place and at the right time can trigger such a domino effect. This may activate the self-corrective forces throughout the primary respiratory system and create changes affecting the whole person.

FLUID SKILLS

As human engineers, as physicians, we are dealing with the most powerful
force within the human body when we learn to use the tidal movements of
body physiology, tidal movements designed by the Master Mechanic.[49]
DR ROLLIN BECKER D.O.

As well as gently working with the patient's tissues, the practitioner can also subtly encourage motion of the patient's fluid systems. According to Dr Sutherland, the longitudinal fluctuation of cerebrospinal fluid (C.S.F.) is the fundamental principle in the craniosacral concept.[50] C.S.F. is like the rechargeable battery fluid of the body, carrying the potency of the Breath of Life. Dr Sutherland referred to this potency as an invisible element carried in the fluid.[51] Wherever C.S.F. goes, so potency also goes, just as energy in the form of heat is carried around in a central heating system.

While the role of cerebrospinal fluid is central to the distribution of potency in the body, other fluids (such as blood, lymph and interstitial fluid) also share this important function. If all the fluid systems are unrestricted in their motion, the ordering principle of the Breath of Life can manifest without obstruction.

Fluid and potency are fundamental intrinsic resources in the patient's physiology which can be employed for encouraging health. They bring increased order and vitality wherever they go. The potency carried in the fluids can be relied upon to provide maximum benefit to areas of disorder. Therefore, by simply facilitating the expression of fluid and potency, inertial patterns can be resolved and the original matrix of health restored, obviating the need for more invasive forms of treatment. There are three common approaches to working with fluids and potency:

1 working with lateral fluctuations of fluid
2 encouraging a V-spread
3 encouraging the longitudinal fluctuation of fluid.

Working with lateral fluctuations

When the longitudinal fluctuation of fluid encounters the resistance provided by an inertial fulcrum, various eccentric patterns of fluid motion may be produced. These eddies, currents and side-to-side motions are referred to as 'lateral fluctuations' (see Chapter 6). Wherever there are lateral fluctuations, the presence of an inertial fulcrum is indicated.

As potency is carried in the fluids, the practitioner's encouragement of lateral fluctuations towards the site of an inertial fulcrum can bring vital resources to the area. This increases the amount of biodynamic potency available to resolve inertial forces.

Lateral fluctuations can be gently exaggerated by the hands, as if pushing a child on a swing, at the start of each pendulate phase of its motion. If an inertial fulcrum is located between the practitioner's hands, the fluid will rebound against this resistance. However, as the potency carried in the fluid starts to have an effect on the fulcrum, its gradual and progressive dissolution may be palpated with each new lateral fluctuation. In many instances this procedure alone is sufficient to sort out an inertial pattern.

Encouraging a V-spread

This approach is used to work with inertial forces held in joints or sutures. It applies two principles of treatment simultaneously: directing potency and fluid towards a site of inertia, while at the same time suggesting a disengagement of bones that have become compressed together.

The practitioner directs potency towards the joint being treated by giving the fluid in the area a subtle nudge towards the inertial fulcrum. This impulse is introduced by one hand placed at a point on the opposite surface of the body. Encouraging fluid and potency towards an immobile joint is like applying some deep penetrating lubricating oil.[52] One patient described how he experienced the sensation of this 'like warm water bringing relief' into his painful arthritic knee. The practitioner also makes a V-shape with two fingers of the other hand. This 'V' is placed either side of the immobile joint (see Figure 7.5). While fluid and potency are directed towards the joint, the practitioner facilitates its disengagement by suggesting a widening of the V-shape in his fingers.

Encouraging longitudinal fluctuation

A clear and vital expression of the natural longitudinal fluctuation of C.S.F. is necessary to distribute potency and its ordering principle throughout the primary respiratory mechanism. The fluctuation of C.S.F. may be gently encouraged along its midline axis in order to increase the availability of potency in the body. This can be done by suggesting a subtle push into the fluid at the start of its inhalation and exhalation phases, helping to encourage its amplitude of motion. Again, this is like pushing a child on a swing. The longitudinal fluctuation of fluid is gradually increased with each gentle push.

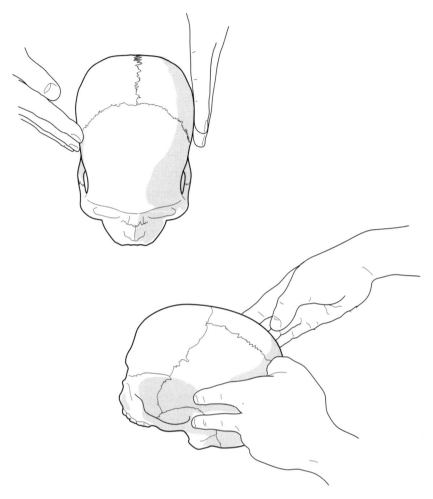

Figure 7.5: V-spread process for the squamosal suture (between temporal and parietal bone)

STILLPOINTS

At the still point of the turning world. Neither flesh nor fleshless;
Neither from nor towards; at the still point, there the dance is,
But neither arrest nor movement. And do not call it fixity,
Where past and future are gathered. Neither movement from
nor towards,
Neither ascent nor decline. Except for the point, the still point,
There would be no dance, and there is only the dance.[53]

T. S. ELIOT

A *stillpoint* is a period of deep physiological rest for the body during which there is a temporary cessation of the cranial rhythmic impulse (C.R.I.). It differs from a 'local stillpoint' which is found at the point of balanced tension, because here a stillness occurs throughout the whole system. As the C.R.I. settles, the inherent fluctuation of cerebrospinal fluid, the flexion/extension and external/internal rotation of tissues come to a point of rest. This kind of 'systemic stillpoint' may last anything from a few seconds to several minutes.

The temporary cessation of the C.R.I. occurs quite naturally from time to time, especially if someone is in a state of good health. It is a rest period during which the body physiology is able to recharge and resource. In fact, a proper balance between stillness and activity is a prerequisite for the manifestation of good health. According to Dr Becker,

> The stillness is that which centres every molecule of being of that living
> body. The body physiology is the outward expression of that stillness. They
> are in total unity, in balanced interchange ... Health is related to a return
> to the freedom of interchange between body physiology and stillness.[54]

However, if stressed or overwhelmed, the body's ability to settle and find stillness may be lost, so recharging cannot take place. This frequently happens with people who suffer from prolonged stress, or who keep pushing themselves and consequently find it hard to slow down. Eventually a diminishing of potency reserves can result, creating a state of exhaustion. Encouraging stillpoints can help reverse this tendency, enabling the patient to let go and find new balance.

During a stillpoint, the body has the opportunity to take up more potency of the Breath of Life and recharge. This is like getting plugged back into the mains and charging up the battery fluid (i.e. cerebrospinal fluid). It is in this stillness that the source of potency or power can be found.[55] When fluid takes up more potency, the expression of the ordering principle of the Breath of Life is facilitated. Our intrinsic biodynamic forces may then have an opportunity to re-organize inertial patterns and encourage an integration of function.

Finding stillness is like letting a glass of muddy water settle. It may seem that the mud and water are inseparable, in the same way that stress or trauma may seem like an inseparable part of our experience. However, if you let the water settle, all the mud goes to the bottom. If you want to drink the water, or even just look through the glass, it's better not to shake the glass. In the same way, there is no need to 'dig up the dirt' in order to find a clarity in mind and body. Furthermore, when the dirt in a muddy pond is given a chance to settle to the bottom, you may even find that lotus flowers grow out of it! As Lao Tzu writes,

Do you have the patience to wait
till your mud settles and the water is clear?
Can you remain unmoving
till the right action arises by itself?[56]

Stillpoints can be facilitated by the practitioner providing a subtle resistance with his hands to either the inhalation or exhalation phase of the C.R.I. The C.R.I. is followed to the end of either phase and then gently invited to stay there by the suggestion of a little back pressure brought into the tissues or fluids. This is commonly done with hand contacts at the occiput, sacrum or feet, but may be facilitated from anywhere in the body. If the patient's physiology is not ready to take up these gentle suggestions, its intelligence is always respected. Nevertheless, as the primary respiratory system usually knows a good thing when it sees it, there is a tendency for these invitations to be accepted.

Compression of the fourth ventricle

One of the most frequently used ways to encourage a stillpoint is from the occiput, encouraging a resting period in the exhalation/extension phase of craniosacral motion. This is called a 'CV4'. CV4 refers to the compression of the fourth ventricle – one of the fluid-filled spaces in the brain, located in front of the occiput (see Figure 3.2, page 41). Many of the vital nerve centres of the body are found in the walls of the fourth ventricle, and their proper functioning is dependent upon the supply of potentized cerebrospinal fluid.

To facilitate a CV4, the practitioner follows the side-to-side narrowing of the occipital bone in its extension phase of craniosacral motion, and then gently encourages a stilling of the tissues at the end of this phase (see Figure 7.6). The narrowing of the occiput happens in synchrony with the exhalation phase of the fourth ventricle, which also narrows as cerebrospinal fluid recedes towards the lower part of the body. Therefore, encouraging extension of the occiput also encourages exhalation of the fourth ventricle. When a stillpoint is reached, the tissues and fluids relax in their exhalation/extension phase. This not only brings deep physiological rest but also encourages potency and its ordering forces to move into the main trunk of the body.

The early cranial osteopaths referred to CV4 as a 'shotgun technique' – just as a shotgun creates a spray of bullets, CV4 produces widespread effects. CV4s are employed whenever potency reserves in the body are low. They also are useful in the treatment of acute fevers, helping fluid drainage in the body, facilitating the removal of wastes, for conditions of stress or anxiety, congestive headaches, sinusitis, digestive disturbances, reproductive disorders and

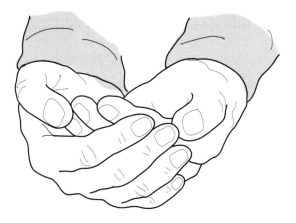

Figure 7.6: Hand position for CV4

for a wide range of other problems. Furthermore, they can also help to clarify the priorities of the primary respiratory mechanism by clearing secondary or peripheral disturbances.[57] In short, there are not many conditions where a CV4 will not be of some benefit.

EV4

Stillpoints can also be facilitated in the inhalation/flexion phase of craniosacral motion. A stillpoint in the inhalation phase is called an 'EV4', which refers to the *expansion of the fourth ventricle*. During an EV4, there is a widening and filling of the ventricles, as fluid and potency move towards the upper part of the body. As well as providing deep physiological rest, EV4s help to distribute any stored-up reserves of potency held in the lower part of the body, facilitating this potency's movement both upwards and outwards to the periphery of the body.

Deep relaxation

As a stillpoint approaches, irregularities such as tremors, a fluttering or pulsations can manifest in the patterns of craniosacral motion. Sometimes the exacerbation of an existing pain or the recurrence of an old familiar pain may surface. It is also at this point that held-in emotions are sometimes experienced. As a stillpoint is reached, lung breathing tends to slow down and everything relaxes. Any pain seems to dissipate and muscle tension subsides. The

patient may take a deep sighing breath, as they let go of the last of any stored-up tension associated with that particular pattern.[58]

A stillpoint is usually accompanied by shifts in mental and emotional processes. Patients
often report that their thinking slows down or even stops. Some experience a state of 'no
thought or doing', just a sense of *being*. This mental state seems very much like the state of
transcendence described in many meditation practices. One patient described it as 'a kind of
roaring silence'.

When a stillpoint is over, the cranial rhythmic impulse naturally restarts its motion, usually
with more fluid drive and a better symmetry. The fluids of the body will have been re-poten-
tized and other physiological functions proceed with greater balance.

Return to the source

Stillness is the doorway to our deeper levels of functioning. After the cranial rhythmic impulse
has settled into stillness, deeper aspects of the primary respiratory system may also settle,
accessing even deeper levels of stillness. In this way we may step into more profound states of
balance and a more direct relationship with our own nature. This is usually experienced as a
dropping down, in stages, into deeper states of relaxation, awareness and integration. In all,
seven levels of stillness have been identified.[59] Each one brings a settling of some further
aspect of our life process:

1 Physical
   *The cranial rhythmic impulse and craniosacral motion become still. The nervous
   system may discharge the effects of trauma.*

2 Emotional
   *The limbic system of the brain (the 'emotional' brain) becomes involved; trapped
   emotions may be discharged.*

3 Psychological
   Life issues become clear as something deeper begins to let go.

4 Heart
   *Any conditioned urges and deeper tendencies of the personality begin to settle.
   Deeper 'karmic' tendencies are released.*

5 Mind
Archetypal energies, talents, ancestral tendencies and deep rooted creative energies are accessed.

6 Spirit
A deep experience of interconnectedness and unity ensues. The patient has a sense of being part of the whole.

7 Source
An indescribable, wordless state beyond duality.

Our source is stillness. Therefore, encouraging stillpoints is the ultimate 're-source', for it puts us back in touch with the place from which the Breath of Life emerges. Within this process of resourcing, an opportunity is provided to create a deeper connection to the well-spring of our inherent health and creativity.[60]

TREATMENT PRACTICALITIES

All technique is correct if it does not interfere with the change emerging, if it allows the patient to become aware of that change and if it promotes continued movement along that path of correction.[61]

R. SMOLEY

The healing crisis

Old symptoms or an intensification of existing ones can sometimes arise during craniosacral treatment, signifying that the body is in a process of re-organization. These acute responses, referred to as a *healing crisis*, may occur as part of the body's attempt to dissipate injury or trauma, and often emerge just prior to the re-establishment of primary respiratory motion. They can be a sign that the resolution of an inertial pattern is close to completion. The 'therapeutic pain' sometimes associated with a healing crisis is even often experienced as 'a good pain', as it is produced when a clarification and clearing of the pattern is taking place.

Sometimes old toxins are eliminated from the body as a result of a re-organization taking place. Occasionally this can manifest as temporary symptoms of diarrhoea, nausea, a cold, acute fever, or skin problems such as rashes or spots. These are part of nature's rebalancing and healing effort. Occasionally, marks appear on the body at the site of an injury being treated. Red marks are typically found in the same place that a bruise or other type of wound was originally experienced. These phenomena arise from a re-creation of the elements present in the original traumatic event.[62] A number of patients have had these red marks appear at the sides of the head, where a forceps injury was sustained during their birth process. These marks soon begin to fade and generally disappear within a few days. If, however, any of these responses becomes too strong, the practitioner can slow down the pace of treatment.

Finding integration

Once an inertial fulcrum has resolved, it can take up to a few days for this change to become integrated throughout the primary respiratory mechanism. This is particularly the case if some age-old or deep-seated pattern has shifted. In the interim, it may feel like being on shifting sands, or as if the carpet has been taken from under your feet. It's therefore not a good idea for the patient to rush around or engage in any strenuous physical activity directly after a treatment. This allows for any changes which have taken place to more easily settle. Furthermore, firmly established inertial patterns may require a number of sessions before they are fully resolved. This may involve experiencing some sensitivity or discomfort before the process of re-organization is complete.

There are a number of therapeutic approaches which can help the patient find balance within any remaining imbalance – the facilitation of stillpoints being one of the most commonly used and effective. Furthermore, the balancing of different tissues that function in harmonic relationship with each other can also help with this process of integration. For example, the sacrum and occiput tend to reflect each other's patterns of primary respiratory motion. If inertia is held in one of these bones, it often affects the other. Therefore, if one bone has been worked with, it is also useful for the functioning of the other to be checked. This can help to integrate the primary respiratory motion of the lower and upper parts of the body. Many bones of the cranium function in a harmonic relationship with bones in the pelvis (see Figure 7.7). The balancing of these harmonically related structures tends to achieve a greater integration of function through the body as a whole.

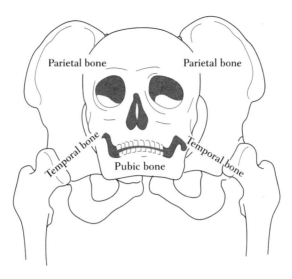

Parietal bone   Parietal bone

Temporal bone   Temporal bone

Pubic bone

Figure 7.7: Harmonic relationship between the cranium and pelvis[63]

Contraindications and warnings!

Like many skills in life (such as driving a car or even crossing the road), craniosacral work is safe as long as it is practised correctly. One of the golden rules of treatment is: at least, do no harm. Any attempt to correct the primary respiratory mechanism by force is not only confrontational, but also potentially harmful. Negative reactions to treatment may occur if techniques are applied without proper consideration of the body's intrinsic ordering principle. The expression of the primary respiratory motion is both prudent and sensitive, and may react to even subtle projections of force (or the intention of force). Even the gentle contacts used in craniosacral work can create problems if misapplied, especially if the patient's available resources of potency are low.

Following the inherent treatment plan of the patient will never lead to adverse reactions. It's true to say, therefore, that there are no universal contraindications to craniosacral work. However, there are contraindications to the application of certain procedures in certain situations. For example, even subtle pressures should not be used on the cranium in conditions such as very high blood pressure, after a recent stroke, intracranial haemorrhage or aneurysm, or in conditions where there is raised fluid pressure in the head. Similarly, caution should be taken after any recent fracture or acute injury. There may also be a risk in working in the region of a malignant tumour, due to the possibility of it spreading. Some practitioners are also wary about applying certain procedures such as CV4 with a patient in the first three months of pregnancy. This is because of the higher risk of miscarriage during this period. However, when a certain approach is contraindicated it is likely that there are others which can be applied safely.

Choosing a therapist

Any therapy with such vast potential for doing good may also do harm if it is practised in the wrong hands. Consequently, patients should be prepared to take personal responsibility, and be discerning about the competence and skill of their practitioner. Craniosacral therapy is unregulated in most countries, and it's an unfortunate fact that there are some people practising this work with only a minimal amount of training. When first making an appointment it is a good idea to enquire about a practitioner's training background. For help with finding a therapist, see the Resource Guide at the end of this book.

Finding the right practitioner is a highly individual matter. No two practitioners are the same. Some may be eminently skilled and qualified, but do not have the right chemistry or 'karma' to help you. Craniosacral work is a subjective science, based on what happens within the particular relationship between practitioner and patient. Each therapeutic relationship is very personal, and to a greater or lesser degree may create the safety to explore patterns of distress. In this respect, a therapist's care and consideration are at least as important as his qualifications. According to spiritual healer Ambrose Worrall, 'The chemistry of compassion is the most powerful factor in ... healing.'[64]

Referrals

The facilities of conventional medical testing are a valuable resource if a diagnosis needs clarification. Furthermore, in many severe cases conventional (allopathic) medicine or surgery may be the most favourable option of treatment. While craniosacral therapy can help a wide variety of patients, different people may need different approaches. For example, the services of a psychotherapist or counsellor may be beneficial for patients with severe emotional and psychological problems. Many cases of severe spinal disc degeneration benefit from the advances of modern surgical intervention. Other alternative therapies such as homeopathy, herbal medicine and acupuncture are also valuable resources. My address book for referrals is perhaps one of the most useful items in my practice.

Nevertheless, craniosacral work can be used in conjunction with other treatments. As Dr Becker commented,

I do not consider myself to be the patient's primary physician ... I still say the patient is the primary physician. Whatever I do is supplementary to whatever other care the patients are getting ... I'm assisting their body to utilize the resources available for their particular health pattern.[65]

Treatment position

Most craniosacral treatments are carried out (at least initially) with the patient lying face-up (supine) on a treatment table. However, side-lying, seated, or face-down (prone) positions are also used. All of these positions are adaptable, according to comfort. Where there is pain, or if the patient is in the latter stages of pregnancy, alternatives can always be used. Disabled patients can be treated while remaining seated in a wheelchair.

Most treatments involve a light contact on the surface of the body, but some procedures involve working from inside the mouth. These 'intra-oral' approaches are commonly used for working with the bones of the face, jaw and palate. In the interests of hygiene, a finger cot or latex glove is always worn in these cases.

Multiple hand treatments

Two practitioners (or sometimes more) can work with the same patient at the same time. The presence of more than one practitioner may amplify the sense of contact and containment felt by the patient. Having a second pair of hands is also very useful for providing physical support if patients move into awkward positions during treatment. Occasionally the practitioner may need assistance from a colleague in encouraging potency towards an inertial fulcrum while working with a tissue pattern. Furthermore, some severe cases respond more quickly when there are several pairs of hands working at the same time.[66]

Self-help

Everything we do can support our health ... or otherwise. Health-building approaches such as taking adequate rest and eating a suitable diet bolster our inner resources and enhance any treatment procedure. Time for fun and a sense of humour also usually work. Health is ultimately the responsibility of each individual. Each person needs to find the things that support them and to follow what suits their constitution. This is a process of self-discovery. If we are able to deal with the origins of diseases, there are possibilities for resolution even in the most intractable of cases. According to an old saying used in Naturopathy, 'There's no such thing as an incurable disease, there are only incurable people.'

Healing can begin as soon as we are able to find a clear relationship to our intrinsic health. One way of forming this relationship is to identify and reconnect with our inner resources (see exercises in Chapter 9). Simply tuning in to the subtle motions produced by the Breath of Life within ourselves is another way to connect with our health (see exercises in Chapter 6). These rhythms are a manifestation of our deepest physiological resources.

Ultimately, all craniosacral treatment is a form of self-help because it always works in co-operation with the self-healing forces of the body. Nevertheless, although the vast majority of health problems are resolved quite naturally without any outside assistance, there will often be difficulties with which our self-healing forces need support. It is then that the practitioner can give a little help along the way. However, this help is not always easy to give oneself, because the hand positions and subtle intentions used in craniosacral work need to be precisely applied. Moreover, it can be difficult to relate clearly to our own inertial patterns. This is because we are often too involved or too close to the source of a problem to discern what may be needed to resolve it.

Having said this, some craniosacral self-treatments can be effective. For example the facilitation of lateral fluctuations of fluid and potency towards the site of an injury can reduce inflammation and bring pain relief. We may also be able to access points or states of balanced tension in patterns of inertia affecting our own tissues. Furthermore, there is an approach to facilitate a CV4 on oneself by laying down and resting the back of the occiput on two tennis balls wrapped together at the end of a sock. If the tennis balls rest either side of the raised bump at the back of the occiput (external occipital protuberance), a stillpoint can be encouraged. However, the advice of a professional practitioner should be sought to clarify if this may be useful in your case.

Frequency of treatment

The frequency of sessions varies according to the condition being treated and the health of each individual. In the average case of a more chronic problem, treatment can be given once or sometimes twice a week until there are some definite signs of improvement. At this point, sessions can be spread out to fortnightly, monthly and then perhaps just some maintenance checks from time to time. An acute problem, however, may need more intensive work at the start of a treatment programme, but then less work long term. While treatment once a week is the average, in some of these cases it may even be given every two to three days until the acute symptoms have subsided. However, these are all generalizations; each case needs to be assessed on its own merits.

An evolutionary process

For shifts in health to occur, the conditions maintaining the problem have to be ripe for change. Creating ripeness for health is an evolutionary process rather than a specific event. In craniosacral work the body is supported to resolve its inertial patterns in a sequential, unfolding manner. Steps one, two, three, four, etc. are taken during this process until there are no more steps to take and healing is complete. The further emergence of health is always built on the basis of previous steps taken. If the foundations for health are not established and we try to trick the body with a drug, an external force, 'mental gymnastics' or posturing, then sooner or later we will fail. The missing steps must be taken for health to be sustained.

RETURN TO WHOLENESS

The philosophical ramifications of this concept are staggering. It means that every one of us matters, that we affect each other in many, many ways never before described. Everything we do matters in the context of the whole. What we do and think affects everyone else. It probably involves planetary consciousness and much broader aspects of humanness than are currently understood.[67]
CARLISLE HOLLAND D.O.

Core levels of functioning

People come for craniosacral treatment for many different reasons and with many motivations. Some know of its benefits for particular physical disorders, others use it to help with stress or psychological difficulties, still others to engender a greater integration of mind, body and spirit. The beauty of this work is that it encompasses all these.

The results of treatment are often remarkable, even when other medical and therapeutic approaches have failed. The depth of craniosacral work is explained by the fact that it works with our most fundamental physiological system, that of primary respiratory motion. This approach has the ability to either by-pass or move through any opinions or mental defences we may carry. It works directly with the wisdom in the body.

Positive transformation

It seems that problems mainly become difficult when they become fragmented in their relationship to the whole. When this relationship is re-established, life and motion resume. Craniosacral treatment provides a clear reflection of physiological and psychological patterns, *and* is able to access the forces of health needed to restore integration. This may be both challenging and at the same time greatly reassuring. As layers of inertial patterning become resolved, a deeper connection to our own nature evolves.

When primary respiratory motion is restored and the original matrix of health re-emerges, clarity and balance return to both body and mind. This brings a reconnection to a profound sense of 'OK-ness'. It is perhaps then that a feeling of 'this is how I really am' can emerge.[68] As a practitioner, this positive process of transformation is always a privilege to witness.

Greater flexibility

The motion of life creates a state of constant change. Our freedom, fluidity and flexibility to accommodate for life's intrinsic movement are in direct relationship to our health and happiness. Craniosacral treatment encourages a greater flexibility of function and enables us to move more easily with the natural rhythms of life. It provides the conditions for a depth of healing to occur, while being sufficiently open so as not to stifle or suppress the infinite possibilities that the innate intelligence within each one of us may wish to bring about. This can be an important part of the realization of our potential on physical, psychological and spiritual levels.

As we undergo a commitment to work with ourselves in this way, our relationship to the body, to our feelings, to our friends or partners, to our work and to life itself can become more open and creative. The path of health and wholeness stretches out before us, all the way towards the Infinite—

Even the hour of our death may send
Us speeding on to fresh and newer spaces,
And life may summon us to newer races.[69]
HERMANN HESSE

8

A HOLISTIC
VIEW

The human body, at peace with itself,

is more precious than the rarest gem.

Cherish your body, it is yours this one time only.

The human form is won with great difficulty,

it is easy to lose.

All worldly things are brief, like lightning in the sky;

This Life you must know as the tiny splash of a raindrop;

a thing of beauty that disappears even as it comes into being .

Therefore set your goal,

Make use of every day and night to achieve it.[1]

TSONG KHAPA

ORIGINS OF DISORDERS

*By concentrating on smaller and smaller fragments of the body, modern
medicine perhaps loses sight of the patient as a whole human being, and
by reducing health to mechanical functioning it is no longer able to deal
with the phenomenon of healing.*[2]
H.R.H. PRINCE CHARLES

From the core of our bodies to the periphery, patterns of inertia may restrict primary respiratory motion and so affect our health. Causes as diverse as physical injury, trauma, poor nutrition, environmental pollution, and genetic and psychological factors can all have their
influence. From the soil to the soul we are a part of life's process and may be subject to its
conditioning forces. In this chapter we will consider the origins of illness and look further at
the important connection between mind, body and spirit.

Physical Trauma

Physical injury is a common cause of inertial patterning in the body. Incidents such as blows,
cuts, falls and accidents create protective contractions in the tissues that may remain long
after the original trauma has passed. As long as our intrinsic resources are unable to deal with
an injury, its effects stay with us. Scars received as a result of tissue damage or surgery may
act as one such site of disturbance. Scars can pull on surrounding tissues and consequently
influence the motion of even distant areas of the body.

Another frequent and significant cause of physical trauma is a difficult birth. We will be looking at this issue in Chapter 10.

Impact of forces

All the muscles, bones, fluids and organs of the body have a certain density. Whenever a
physical force is encountered, it meets the resistance provided by these tissues. As the biokinetic energy of an incoming force meets this resistance, its velocity slows down and eventually reaches a particular place where it comes to a stop (see Figure 8.1). If the force is very
strong, the tissues can suffer damage or breakage along the way. The point at which the biokinetic energy of a physical force stops is where it may remain lodged if the body's intrinsic
forces are unable to dissipate it. This place of energy entrapment is often located some

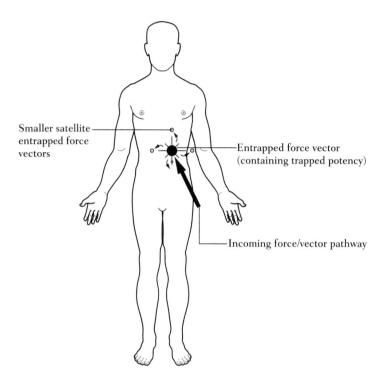

Smaller satellite
entrapped force
vectors

Entrapped force vector
(containing trapped potency)

Incoming force/vector pathway

Figure 8.1: Formation of entrapped force vector

distance from the actual site of impact. Powerful kinetic forces may sometimes even pass right through the tissues, forming a fulcrum of organization outside the body.

Entrapped force vector

If the body's capacity to dissipate a traumatic force is overwhelmed, the incoming energy is treated as a kind of foreign object. As such, a contraction forms in the surrounding tissues, helping to wall it off. This response minimizes the effect on nearby tissues. In time, tissues become more permanently organized in relationship to the trapped biokinetic force, adopting a habitual pattern of contraction. This process is similar to how the lungs wall off an infection of tuberculosis bacteria, forming a calcified cyst.[3] Consequently, a walled-off area of biokinetic potency is produced around which primary respiratory motion then has to organize.

This particular type of inertial fulcrum is called an *entrapped force vector* or *energy cyst*.[4] The term 'vector' refers to the pathway that the kinetic energy of a trauma takes as it enters the body (see Figure 8.1).

This vector pathway may be in a straight line or bent, depending on the angle at which the force enters the body. If the body moves at the time of a traumatic accident (which is frequently the case), the vector pathway tends to bend as it passes through the moving tissues. This causes the vector pathway to become curved.

If the force vector meets something solid, such as a bone, it can sometimes splinter into different branches, forming satellite energy cysts. This may result in the formation of various smaller inertial fulcrums (see Figure 8.1).

An entrapped force vector may result in the formation of tissue adhesions, disturbances in fluid motion, poor circulation, a build-up of toxicity and nerve irritation. Franklyn Sills notes, 'These protective responses may be useful at the initial time of the experience, but can become locked into the system as deeply-ingrained protective patterning.'[5] A number of practitioners have also noted a correspondence between the sites of energy entrapments and the development of tumours. Dr John Upledger observes,

> The body adapts somewhat to the presence of energy cysts, but in the
> process ideal function is compromised, interference waves are produced,
> normal electrical conductivity of involved body tissues is reduced and the
> flow of energy along acupuncture meridians is obstructed. All of this saps
> body energy and creates pain and dysfunction.[6]

Interference waves

The 'interference waves' referred to by Dr Upledger are three-dimensional patterns of energy emanating from the site of an active disturbance. They are like the ripples of water produced when a stone is thrown into a pond. These waves can be sensed by palpation as arcs of energy radiating out from the site of an entrapped force vector. They may be noticed if the practitioner maintains a light and airy quality to his perception. The closer to the fulcrum of disturbance, the faster and stronger these waves become. Therefore, by following the pattern of interference waves all the way back to their source it is possible to locate the site of an entrapped force vector.

Emotional coupling

If any strong emotions are experienced at the time of a trauma, they may become coupled together with the entrapped force vector. For example, if anger or fear is experienced when a force vector enters, this emotion may become retained in the body, as part of the pattern. Emotions can be an important element in both organizing and maintaining the inertial fulcrum (see The Mind–Body Continuum, page 196).

Nutrition and Diet

The food we eat provides essential ingredients for the development of healthy tissue and plays an important role in building up our resources of vitality. However, poor nutrition leads to weakness of the tissues and a build-up of toxicity, which can influence the functioning of the primary respiratory system. Not only is the intake of a well-balanced diet needed to furnish the cells of the body with health, but so is the proper absorption of these nutrients by the digestive tract and the elimination of any wastes. The ability of the digestive organs to express primary respiratory motion is imperative for these functions – absorbing nutrients, getting rid of wastes – to be efficiently carried out.

Build-up of toxicity

If the organs of elimination (mainly the bowel and skin) become overloaded, then waste products and toxins cannot be discarded effectively. These are then stored in the body, which may lead to the development of toxic build-up. As far as the body is concerned, this toxicity is another kind of biokinetic force which its intrinsic forces of health have to try to deal with. Some waste products may find their way into the connective tissues, joints, muscles and fluids of the body for storage, causing a lack of motility, tissue adhesions and the development of inertial patterns. A variety of degenerative conditions such as arthritis, disorders of the digestive organs or cancer may result.[7] A build-up of toxicity can also occur due to factors like food processing, chemical additives, pesticides, over- or under-cooking and the use of drugs.

Frequently, a lack of potency can be palpated in the tissues of someone who eats a lot of junk food or who is a smoker or heavy drinker. In such cases, craniosacral motion is often expressed with a quality of sluggishness or congestion. When this type of inertial pattern is resolved, the toxic substances which became stored in the body can be eliminated. This often leads to a healing crisis as these substances are dissipated from the tissues. In a number of cases I have treated, skin eruptions, acute colds, fever or diarrhoea have followed the resolution of toxic inertial fulcrums.

Effects of drugs

Drugs are frequently a source of nutritional imbalance in the body. Apart from the fact that many commonly prescribed drugs destroy certain vitamins and minerals, they are also a major source of toxicity. In fact there is no such thing as a drug without a side-effect. Any substance which artificially produces a specific effect on certain tissues or systems has to be accommodated for by the body. Even if these side-effects are tolerated or dissipated, the balancing adjustments necessary can put a considerable strain on the intrinsic resources of the primary respiratory system.

The effects of drugs can sometimes be clearly palpable in the expressions of primary respiratory motion, particularly in the quality of fluid fluctuation. Antibiotics tend to cause a vibration and jumpiness in the fluids, anti-depressants a quality of sluggishness. The long-term use of painkillers causes a dullness and general dissociation. Anaesthetic drugs are frequently palpated within the fluids as a rapid quivering and coldness, as often arises when the after-effects of surgery are being processed.

Recreational drugs can also have a profound effect. Cannabis, for example, interferes with the ability of fluids to take up the ordering principle of the Breath of Life and gives primary respiratory motion a muddied and disorganized quality. For this reason it can be quite difficult to treat people who use recreational drugs. Trying to build up potency resources in some of these cases is a bit like pouring water into a bucket full of holes. When drugs start to dissipate from the tissues during treatment, the qualities mentioned (e.g. disorganization) are sometimes experienced as noticeable sensations by the patient. Not infrequently, drugs can also be smelled or tasted as they are dissipated.

A suitable diet

Generally speaking, a healthy diet contains all the essential nutrients taken in the proper combinations. The best nutritional value is provided by foods grown in uncontaminated soil, containing as few additives and chemicals as possible and free from excessive processing. Ideally, a high proportion of fresh, living foods should be eaten. These foods, consisting primarily of whole grains, seeds, sprouts, nuts, fresh fruits and vegetables, are rich in nutrients and contain plenty of vital force which helps to build the foundations for health.

The details of what constitutes a healthy diet are beyond the scope of this book, but as this is usually an individual matter, the reader can make further explorations simply by listening to their own body. Let your body tell you what it does and doesn't need. Pay attention to how it responds to what you eat. Take time to feel the sensations created by your food, and let these sensations be your guide. For example, do you feel any discomfort or bloating after meals, or do you get tired easily? You can then explore what kind of diet is more suitable for you by experimenting with other foods. It's far better to trust the wisdom of the body than to make rules or create fads which may or may not be applicable to your individual constitutional requirements.

Environmental Effects

We are an integral part of the world in which we live; our state of health is intimately related to the conditions which surround us. Both our inner and outer worlds need to be in balance for optimal health to result. However, we may live in an environment where this balance is hard to find. Water, food and air may all contain levels of pollutants that have a devitalizing affect on the body. For those (like myself) who live in a large city, we may go for long periods of time never seeing much beyond the next building. It is easy to then lose sight of natural horizons, as a perceptual contraction habitually sets in and a sense of perspective is forgotten. Almost wherever we are, we may be subject to the fast and chaotic influences of modern life, or to other environmental factors such as changes in the weather, or excessive ultra-violet and electromagnetic radiations. Furthermore, environmental influences such as social pressures, family tensions and relationship problems can also have their impact.

Building health

It seems a fairly common experience that external stresses have the greatest impact when our health is already at a low ebb. While nothing beats living in a healthy environment, our inner resources may nevertheless be facilitated to offer greater resilience against harmful influences. Taking the responsibility to be discriminating about what we eat, getting out into nature when we can, exercising and taking adequate rest are all important. Craniosacral treatment, which can access our intrinsic resources of health, can be valuable in helping to build up constitutional strength and so provide benefit even in adverse environmental conditions. At a fundamental level, our intrinsic health is available 24 hours a day, whatever the circumstances.[8]

Hereditary Factors and Genetics

Certain tendencies to ill-health can be passed down from generation to generation. These tendencies are inherited via the genetic 'building blocks' in cells, called DNA. However, now that the mapping of the entire set of human genes has been completed, it has been discovered that they are far less complex than originally thought. The human genetic code shows that we carry little more genetic information than mice, and barely twice as much as tiny fruit flies. Consequently, many scientists have concluded that genes are only *part* of the story in the development of inherited tendencies.

Genetic predispositions do not necessarily mean that we have to suffer from the same problems as our ancestors. As individuals, we are always factors in the equation. According to Eastern systems of medicine there are three core energies converging to form a human being at the moment of conception: the life-force of the mother, the life-force of the father, and the life-force of the incarnating baby. The interplay of all three of these energies has an influence on the constitutional development of the body. If the expression of our own basic life-force is unhindered, it can override tendencies inherited from our parents.

Our options

Furthermore, life is not static; even if there are inherited problems, the expression of our core energies can still be strengthened. I have never come across a case where there is no room for improvement. The presence of our intrinsic health goes deeper than genetics.[9] Genetics can be seen as just a mechanism through which the ordering principle of the Breath of Life carries out its activities. In this age of genetic manipulation, it's easy to lose sight of this deeper intelligence at work.

Although certain inherited predispositions may be present, they often require a certain set of conditions in order to actually manifest as illness. For example, asthma (usually considered to be an inherited illness) often only develops when patterns of inertia affect the motion of the lungs, chest or diaphragm, or when potency resources in the body are low. Similarly, acute attacks of hay fever are often triggered when the cranial nerves which supply the sinuses and tear ducts are irritated. Craniosacral treatment is often able to facilitate the resolution of these underlying conditions.

Mental and Emotional Influences

In many traditional forms of medicine, the body and mind are viewed as inseparable aspects of the same human being. However, now they are usually falsely separated and treated accordingly. Nevertheless, when all the forces that condition our health are considered, the role of the psyche is the most formatively powerful of them all. It is the factor which governs our actions, posture, tensions, diet and many of our responses to life's experiences. In the words of H. H. the Dalai Lama, 'At a deep level mind and body are non-dual.'[10]

The effects of physical trauma, environmental stresses and even hereditary predispositions may all be influenced by the mind. Furthermore, strong emotions or fixed attitudes can act as important fulcrums around which we function. These psychological fulcrums may underpin the physical manifestation of inertia and be critical factors to address in the treatment of disease. To treat the body without considering the role of the psyche is akin to removing dents from a car, while ignoring the ability of the driver.

THE MIND–BODY CONTINUUM

The mind is chief.
All things are mind made.
You are what you think,
having become what you thought.[11]
THE BUDDHA

The mind and body are in continuous and intimate relationship until the day we die. 'Our feelings and attitudes very directly affect the way we hold ourselves, move, breathe and grow.'[12] Consequently, the body is a clear reflector of the person within. Its tone, posture, proportions, tensions, motility, movements, rhythms and vitality all express this relationship.[13] We embody our joys and our suffering.

The body tells a story

The body never lies – it forms itself around who we are inside. If we carry our head low, have tight shoulders, a collapsed chest and walk with a heavy step, these can all reflect feelings of weakness and resignation. In contrast, if our head is carried upright, our shoulders are straight and flexible, our chest is breathing openly and we walk with a springy step, these indicate both confidence and vitality.[14] If we hold ourselves in the world in a certain way due to our beliefs, fears and emotions, the very tissues will take a form that supports this state of mind.

Our physical and psychological traumas as well as our thoughts, feelings and character are reflected in the way our bodies are structurally patterned. The imprints of *any* overwhelming experiences remain held in the body in the form of inertia, fixed there by the inability to access the resources to resolve them, so affecting the expression of our intrinsic health. As Marilyn Ferguson remarks, 'Over the years our bodies become walking autobiographies that tell strangers and friends alike of the major and minor stresses of our lives.'[15] Our body language is the true universal 'Esperanto'.[16]

How cells register feelings

Nowadays, it is becoming more accepted by medical researchers that thoughts and feelings have a direct effect on the functioning of the body. 'Stress' has become linked to a diverse range of diseases including stomach ulcers, cancer, skin problems, backache and infertility. In the field of *psycho-neuroimmunology* (PNI), a number of mechanisms have now been identified through which the mind can influence the body. Previously unrecognized communication networks between the nervous, hormonal and immune systems have been discovered, providing a link between our psychological states and the way in which the response to disease is activated. These mechanisms translate psychological experience into physiological function.

Researchers have noticed that patients suffering from severe depression have higher levels of the hormone *cortisol* circulating in their blood. Cortisol is secreted by the adrenal glands when the body is under stress. However, cortisol also inhibits the activity of the immune system, diminishing its ability to combat disease. It would therefore follow that stress or states of depression have the tendency to lead to illness.

Furthermore, a communication network has been discovered which allows for a two-way transfer of messages between the nervous and immune systems. Nerve endings have been found in some tissues of the immune system, enabling them to directly communicate with the nervous system. These connections disprove previously-held beliefs that the immune system functions independently.

It has also been discovered that the immune cells which help the body to fight infection, called *lymphocytes*, have receptors on their surface able to receive substances such as hormones and neurotransmitters.[17] This links the activity of immune cells with these chemical messengers used by the hormonal and nervous systems. The functioning of lymphocytes, and therefore of the immune response, can be strongly influenced by the brain via the release of hormones and neuro-transmitters. It was also found that lymphocytes produce chemicals called *lymphokines*. These chemicals are capable of transmitting messages back to the brain, so enabling the brain to monitor the activity of lymphocytes and provide a two-way feedback mechanism between these systems.

Amazingly, lymphocytes can also produce hormones able to regulate the activity of the nervous system. This discovery provides another link between the functioning of the immune system and the nervous and hormonal systems. As brain activity is closely related to psychological experience, these findings explain some of the pathways by which mind and body influence each other. In this new understanding, the immune system may even be regarded as an extension of the nervous system, helping it to regulate the inner balance of the body.

Expectations and beliefs

In 1975, Drs Robert Ader and Nicholas Cohen at the University of Rochester School of Medicine and Dentistry discovered that the immune response of rats can be conditioned according to previous experience and expectations, rather like Pavlov's dogs.[18] They conducted a series of experiments in which they paired saccharin-sweetened drinking water with a drug that suppresses the activity of the immune system.[19] Astonishingly, they found that if rats were subsequently given saccharin water alone (without the drug) their immune response was suppressed just as if they were receiving the drug. This so-called *placebo* effect is indicative of the strong effect that beliefs and expectations can have on the functioning of the immune system, and therefore on the body's ability to respond to disease.

Other interesting research was carried out in the cardiac ward of a major American hospital with patients suffering from angina. Angina is a condition in which arteries supplying the heart become restricted, producing acute chest pain. A drug called *digitalis* (traditionally a derivative of the foxglove plant) is known to help with the acute symptoms of an angina attack. Once this drug is administered it generally brings fast relief. In this experiment, 50 per cent of patients who suffered from an acute angina attack were given digitalis, and the other 50 per cent were given a placebo. Even though the second group were given sugar tablets, a significantly high proportion responded favourably and their symptoms subsided.

However, what was even more interesting was that half of the doctors who prescribed the placebo knew that they were doing so, while the other half thought that they were giving their patients the real drug. Surprisingly, the patients who received a placebo from doctors under the impression that they were prescribing the real drug responded much better than the patients who received a placebo from doctors who knew what they were prescribing. So, not only was the belief of the *patient* significant in their response, but so was the confidence of the *doctor*.

The implication of these experiments is that patients who receive treatment from doctors who have a positive outlook on their treatment seem to perform better than patients whose doctors don't believe in what they're doing. Such is the power of the mind! In conventional medicine these placebo effects are usually treated as some kind of inconvenient and negative statistical aberration. However, if the power of the mind can be skilfully harnessed in the therapeutic process, then the possibilities for cure are vastly increased.

Experiences become fixed

From an early age the structural patterning of the body begins to form under the influence of our mental and emotional states. Inertial fulcrums in the tissues frequently develop in relationship to fixed psychological states. In turn, the feelings themselves can become imprisoned within contracted tissues and so become even more 'set in their ways'. Such *psychosomatic* patterns influence our physiological functioning and give us our unique and personally identifiable characteristics of mind and body. Ida Rolf illustrates this point:

> An individual experiencing temporary fear, grief or anger, all too
> often carries in his body an attitude which the world recognises as an out-
> ward manifestation of that particular emotion. If he persists in this drama-
> tisation or consistently re-establishes it, thus forming what is ordinarily
> referred to as a 'habit pattern', the muscular arrangement becomes set.
> Materially speaking, some muscles shorten and thicken, others are
> invaded by connective tissue, still others become immobilised by
> consolidation of the tissue involved. Once this has happened, the physical
> attitude is invariable; it is involuntary; it can no longer be changed
> basically by taking thought or even by mental suggestion. Such setting of
> a physical response also establishes an emotional pattern. Since it is not
> possible to establish a free flow through the physical flesh, the subjective
> emotional tone becomes progressively more limited and tends to remain in
> a restricted, closely defined area. Now what that individual feels is no
> longer an emotion, a response to an immediate situation, henceforth he
> lives, moves and has his being in an attitude.[20]

An open mind

Research by Dr Pritbin at Stanford University even indicates that habitual mental patterns can create neural grooves in the cortex of the brain. These findings give a whole new meaning to the phrases 'having a one-track mind' or 'fixed ideas'. Thought patterns become literal anatomical grooves in the brain, perhaps also influencing the way in which the central nervous system is able to express its motility. In my experience, an open mind is reflected by an open head – that is, one that is relatively free of resistance to the expressions of primary respiratory motion. A tightness within the cranial and facial movements is often noticeable with people who have a fixed attitude and a closed mind. According to an old African proverb, 'All that is in the heart is written in the face.'

Reflected in the tides

At a deep level of functioning, the rhythmic motions produced by the Breath of Life are a clear and accurate barometer of mental and emotional processes. A lack of primary respiratory motion in different parts of the body may reflect particular feelings which have become associated with the function of these tissues. For example, the mouth may relate to feelings we have about receiving nourishment, and the throat with self-expression. The lower back may be connected to feelings of support, and the pelvis with sexuality and grounding. Dr John Upledger describes a common pattern of compressed tissues found in patients who suffer from depression: This pattern consists of a triad of inertial tissues at the *spheno-basilar junction*, the *cranial base* and the *lumbosacral junction*.[21] It seems that when the motion at these important junctions becomes restricted, the flow of life's creative forces gets significantly dammed up.

A clear, vital and smooth quality to the phases of primary respiratory motion may be palpated where peace, happiness and joy are present. In many cases where there is sadness, fear or despondency, qualities of sluggishness, restriction or dullness may result. A lack of confidence may manifest as hesitancy, anxiety as shakiness. Some practitioners even draw a correspondence between mental and emotional states and the way the tissues express their rhythmic movements of flexion and extension. Craniosacral flexion (with side-to-side expansion) can be associated with action and extroversion, while the extension phase corresponds with passivity or introversion. According to how the body's tissues have become patterned, a person may be predominantly a flexion-type or an extension-type. A predominance of either flexion or extension in the rhythms of craniosacral motion may be found with its associated mental state. However, these are broad generalizations and do not necessarily reflect what is happening within any given individual.

Circular feedback

Any fragmentation of primary respiratory motion correlates with a fragmentation of function affecting the whole person. Physiological patterns and emotional experience are mutually perpetuating. The influence of mind on matter and of matter on mind appears to be a kind of circular feedback system, with each one affecting the other. As psychological experiences become embodied, the fixed body patterns then influence our experience. What we call consciousness and our physical expression are a continuum. It is only when this mind-emotion-body continuum comes into a harmonious alignment that the Breath of Life is able to manifest with integration and balance, and optimal health is the result.

Emotional experience

Earlier we noted how physical injuries can become coupled with particular emotions. As we are not just physical beings, the way that we respond to any experience in life naturally involves the mind as well. The mind is a part of everything that we do. If tissues contract in a protective response to stress or trauma, the thoughts and feelings that we have at the time can become an element within that contraction. In particular, strong and overpowering emotions such as terror or despair tend to actively contribute towards the development of inertia, and can then play a significant part in its maintenance. A fulcrum can thus comprise tissues, fluids and potencies which have become restricted, together with entrapped emotions, feeling tones, self-views and beliefs. Dr Viola Frymann concludes that, 'It becomes apparent that there is no such thing as a purely physical problem, an emotional problem or a mental problem.'[22]

Helen's story

Helen was a remarkably young 78-year-old woman who came for treatment after receiving a whiplash injury during a car accident. She was a stylish and active person who had not lost any of her elegance despite the advancing years. Another car had hit hers from behind, just a few weeks after she had completed a previous course of craniosacral work for neck pain. All her old symptoms had since returned. In addition she was experiencing chest pains where she had been hit by the steering wheel. She was 'furious' about the accident and explained that she would get annoyed every time she felt the pain.

Helen felt better immediately after the first couple of treatments, but each time her symptoms soon came back. At the third visit she became visibly agitated whilst my hands were gently placed over her chest. Her eyes were open and furtively looking around. I felt that her upper ribs were restricted in their primary respiratory motion and there was a strong pull towards her back, probably sustained from the force of the steering wheel hitting her. Although there were some tentative moves towards a resolution, the process still felt incomplete.

By Helen's next visit her chest pains had slightly improved, but the neck pain persisted as before. While my hands were at the base of her skull, the tissues in her neck went into strong contraction and shutdown. Helen declared that she was fed up and deeply worried that she might never be pain-free again as a result of the accident. She found these feelings hard to accept, as she had always thought of herself as someone able to cope with difficulties. A few reluctant tears appeared in her eyes.

With a little support, Helen started to give herself permission to explore her feelings of vulnerability. Slowly she began to let go, and became progressively more weepy. As a result the remaining tension in her chest was able to subside, craniosacral motion restarted in her neck and a much fuller sense of primary respiratory motion could be felt throughout her body. When I saw her again two weeks later, Helen's symptoms had dramatically improved. It seems that once the emotional fulcrum – which was an integral part of her distress – had resolved, the healing of her trauma could progress.

Frozen experiences

While to some extent suffering may be a natural and unavoidable part of our lives, it can become trapped in the body as a *frozen experience* if we are unable to let it go. Both the retained physical and emotional conditioning then remain in our everyday lives. This frequently occurs at an unconscious level.

Our previous experiences may colour our response to any new stresses that we face. These conditioned responses mean that we are no longer able to see situations for what they really are, but only in terms of what they trigger in us. The way we deal with new situations can then be like a record which is stuck, as we follow the same pre-set and confined reactions. When 'our buttons get pressed', we act in ways that have more to do with the past experience than our immediate situation. We become trapped by the past instead of just being open to the present. Examples of this are: an emotionally pressurized young man who has to escape on his motorbike and head for open spaces whenever faced with demands, a young child abandoned as a baby who screams when left alone, and the victim of sexual abuse who freezes whenever she is approached with intimacy. The world is always seen according to the tint of the glasses through which we are looking. Moreover, these psycho-physical fulcrums fragment the expression of our original intention of health.

Over-reactions

Previous traumas may sometimes become restimulated with even the slightest provocation. If there is a lot of energy or potency dammed up behind one of these inertial patterns, our reactions can be all the more powerful. If, in addition, strong emotions are coupled with the pattern, we may be like a time bomb waiting to go off. When these traumas become restimulated, the emotional reaction will probably be way 'over the top'. The development of over-sensitivity and frequent emotional outbursts are common symptoms of this. In these examples, the present-time situation, rather than being the cause, is simply like 'the straw which breaks the camel's back'.

Role of connective tissues

While inertial patterns which have a psychological origin may manifest anywhere in the body, the connective tissues seem to play an especially significant role in storing these experiences as *tissue memory*. In particular the fascial network of the body often provides a medium for the storage of trapped emotional energy. For example, withheld anger may manifest as a restricted diaphragm and tightness around the solar plexus, which perhaps then leads to digestive problems and back pain. This type of pattern is frequently held in place by the inter-connections of fascia, which link different regions of the body. The inertial forces holding this kind of contraction in place can usually be resolved when points or states of balance are accessed in the fascial tissues. When this occurs it's not unusual for any associated emotions to come to the surface.

Rings of a tree

The pioneering psychotherapist Dr Wilhelm Reich wrote about how our tissues become contracted to help deaden feelings which are too painful to deal with. Tissues become organized in layers of armouring which serve to protect our vulnerable feelings. He referred to the self-protective buffer against feeling emotions as *character armour*, and of its manifestation in the tissues as *body armour*.[23] Body psychologist Dr Ken Dychtwald comments,

> *Body armour, the physical counterpart of character armour, served the function of encasing the person in his own protective muscular shell. This shell not only kept out harmful or painful stimuli but also served to limit the experience of fearful and painful emotions from within.*[24]

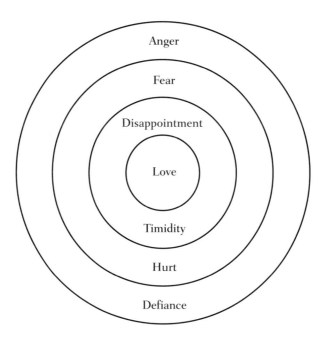

Figure 8.2: Rings of experience

This emotional and structural layering can be organized like the rings of a tree, which develop according to age and experience. For example, an experience of defiance and anger may cover fear and hurt, which in turn cover timidity and disappointment. At the very core of these rings of patterned experience is our basic health, our original matrix and the core emotion of OK-ness and love (see Figure 8.2). Each layer of these feelings may have a structural architecture in the body. The outer layer may be stiff and inflexible, protecting and covering withdrawal and contraction, which in turn cover a sense of collapse in the tissues. Underlying this there is essential health and vitality. Letting go of these structural patterns in the body can be likened to peeling away the layers of an onion (which also sometimes brings tears!). In this process, each layer of fragmented experience needs to be integrated before the next can be dealt with.

Patients' 'languaging'

I have often found it very revealing to listen to the way in which people describe their symptoms. The words or phrases we use can often point to the underlying psychological fulcrums which organize our patterns. For example, we may describe something or someone as 'a pain in the neck', or not be able to 'face' something, and consequently suffer from neck tension. We may talk about a situation that 'makes us sick' or that we 'cannot stomach', or we may not have 'the gall'. We may be 'put out of joint' or 'carry something on our shoulders'. One patient with acutely contracted lower back muscles described how he was feeling 'held back' in his life. When I asked a patient who had diarrhoea why she didn't talk to her husband about some of the unhappiness she was holding inside, she replied that she 'didn't have the guts'! Another patient who had suffered repeated episodes of sexual abuse as a child had developed an acute rash around her pelvis. When she was being treated the memory of her father approaching came vividly into her mind and she described him as 'being all over me like a rash'!

Sometimes the way things are described can be amusing as well as revealing. I was taking the case history of a divorced middle-aged woman who came for treatment because she was in pain with sciatica which radiated down to her left buttock. When I asked her what was happening in her life, she replied that she was feeling 'rather left behind'! Another patient described the pains down his leg as a problem with his 'psychiatric' (sciatic) nerve! While taking the case history of a man who had come for treatment of a low back problem, he told me that he was born with an undescended right testicle. When he was 10 years old he went into hospital for an operation to help this testicle descend. However, after the surgery it moved even further up into his pelvis. He described the operation as 'a right balls up'![25]

Tissue memory

To summarize, our emotions, attitudes and body patterns reflect, enhance and maintain each other.[26] Emotional experiences and psychological beliefs shape the body's tissues, and this in turn predisposes us to particular emotions and set attitudes. Patterns of mind and body become mutually sustaining.

If there is no inertia present, thoughts, feelings and sensations can flow freely through the body without attachment or obstruction. However, overpowering or repetitive experiences are physiologically stored in the form of tissue memory. As Ken Dychtwald remarks, the body becomes 'a storehouse for emotions and beliefs'.[27] At a fundamental level, tissue memories are maintained by trapped inertial forces (from physical and psychological causes). As long as these forces remain in the body, experiences keep cycling in recurrent patterns without getting resolved.

Consequently, an inertial fulcrum may be comprised of a number of different layers. It may involve a contraction which affects the motion of tissues and fluids, feelings and beliefs which are associated with that contraction, and inertial forces which hold the pattern in place.

The psychological aspects of a pattern are often the key elements maintaining it. These trapped emotions and attitudes may only dissipate when we find the resources, the space and the skills to let them go. Creating the conditions for this to happen is the essential point in treatment.

BODY AND ENERGY

My notion of the life force doesn't arise from complex metaphysical or philosophical doctrines. It's based on simple observation and a workaday understanding completely accessible to anyone.[28]

ROBERT FULFORD D.O.

The nature of life

All life is composed of energy. In modern physics, the electron microscope has enabled us to view particles so minute that the boundary between what is called physical matter and energy is now difficult to define.[29] Essentially, matter can be seen as a mass of vibrating energy which has become crystallized into a particular form. Furthermore, this energy is not static. It is part of a dynamic process, with cycles of birth, decay, death and regeneration occurring at every moment. Consequently, our physical selves (and our physical universe) are not as stable or real as perhaps we might think.

Creation is a constant process, not just something that happened a few billion years ago or at the time of our conception. The cells of the body are continually changing, in ever-shifting cycles. Every day we make about 150 million new cells. The cells in the digestive organs live an average of about three months, while muscle cells live for 14 months. The cells that line the stomach will probably have gone through two generations by the time you've finished reading this chapter. Bone cells live for up to six years. By the end of seven years you've made a whole new body![30] Nothing is fixed. The body's form is something that has become arranged in a certain way at a particular moment in time. This means that in each moment we possess great potentialities for healing and positive change.

What is at the basis of this process? This, of course, is the *big* question! While the mystery of life remains, one thing is clear: there is an intelligent force which operates throughout creation. This much, at least, we can observe and experience. The presence of a fundamen-

tal and intelligent force becomes apparent if we simply look at the staggering degree of organization in the natural world. This fundamental force is a universal principle, which in craniosacral work is called the Breath of Life. The unique expression of this universal principle
produces the distinctive rhythmic motions of fluid and tissue found in each person. Without
the organizing forces of the Breath of Life there would be no health, no life and no motion.
As Franklyn Sills explains,

> Creation unfolds in each of us, moment to moment. Creation is
> constantly arising in the present. As every moment arises and passes,
> there is a moment of creation. And it is creation which is centering
> our experience. It is that inherent intention and organization of a
> human being, just in this very moment, as an expression of the
> creativity of the universe, which supports our experience of life.[31]

Our life-force

The concept that there is an intelligent, vital force at the basis of life goes back for thousands of years. A balanced flow of energy as a prerequisite to good health is recognized in
various cultures around the world. From Asia to Africa, Australia to the Americas this knowledge of a vital force has long been incorporated into the healing arts. It is only in modern
Western culture that vital force has become divorced from medicine (as well as spirit from
matter). Certainly, it's a sobering thought that a vitalistic approach to medicine is recognized in about 80 per cent of the world, while a purely materialistic approach is practised in
only 20 per cent.[32]

Nevertheless, the very foundations of medical practice in the West was built upon an
understanding of our vital force as a therapeutic medium. In ancient Greece, Hippocrates
(the father of modern medicine) perceived this force as the 'healing power of nature'. In
17th-century Europe, the great alchemist and doctor, Paracelcus, emphasized the importance of dynamic forces of the natural world operating in harmony with the body. In the
18th century, Viennese-born physician Franz Mesmer described the theory of 'animal
magnetism'. Mesmer wrote about a fluid-like energy surrounding and permeating all life
forms. He asserted that the human body had poles and other properties similar to magnets,
and that through this magnetic medium one person could act upon another to trigger a
process of healing.

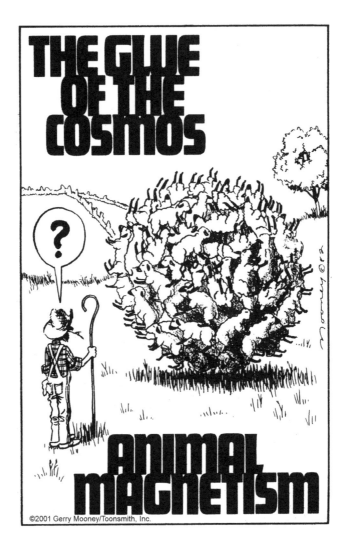

Figure 8.3: Animal Magnetism (cartoon by Gerry Mooney)

Many practitioners now recognize the presence of other subtle bodies of energy which underlie and permeate the physical body. In the book *Philosophy of Natural Therapeutics*, Jocelyn Proby explains,

> *The physical body ... is not the whole man and perhaps not really the essential man at all ... The physical body ... is part of a much larger whole and is linked to other bodies which act upon it and are acted upon by it ...*

*The physical body is subject to the influence of energies which
are brought to bear on it and flow into it from both these other
bodies and from outside.*[33]

These subtle bodies extend beyond the confines of the physical body, radiating out and around as an energy field or 'aura'. It is probable that we respond to these fields of energy without necessarily being aware of it. For example, someone may come and sit behind you on a bus or train, and you may feel a particular response even though you haven't actually seen them. Maybe there's a discomfort or an attraction as they enter your field, even when no contact is made through any of the five senses.

In 1935, Northrup and Burr developed the theory that there is an electromagnetic basis to all living creatures. They concluded that all species are controlled and maintained by an underlying electromagnetic field, which they called the 'L'- or 'life-field'. They likened the L-field to a mould which holds together the cells of the body and vitalizes it. This theory shows remarkable similarities to the role taken by the biodynamic potency of the Breath of Life, recognized by craniosacral practitioners. When a person dies, the L-field or life-force withdraws and the body cells start to disintegrate. Burr stated that the source of disease and imbalance lay first and foremost in disturbances in our energy fields, and that these must be recognized for accurate diagnosis and treatment.[34]

Primary energy

Let's consider some of the different layers of energy present in the human system. In the craniosacral concept, the Breath of Life is seen as the essential ordering force of mind and body. The Breath of Life has been called *primary energy*, for it is our most undifferentiated form of energy, like the reference beam of a hologram.[35] The notion of a primary energy system is also acknowledged in some other forms of medicine. For example, Dr Randolph Stone, the founder of Polarity Therapy, referred to this basic force as a *neuter essence*. Like Dr Sutherland, he considered it to be a fundamental ordering principle.[36] A similar idea is found in traditional systems of medicine in Asia. As Franklyn Sills points out,

In Chinese Medicine the emphasis is on the balance of chi *and the
potency of* jing *in the body. Interestingly,* jing *or 'essence' is similarly
sensed to be an inherent ordering principle in the human body intimately
related to its fluid systems. In Ayurvedic medicine there is a similar
concept in which* ojas *is sensed to be an essential ordering energy which
again manifests in the fluid systems of the body at a cellular level. Finally,*

*in the Tibetan system of medicine it is traditionally experienced to be
located along the central axis of the body and within the cerebrospinal
fluid and central nervous system.*[37]

Elemental energy

Primary energy then differentiates into various layers of *elemental* energy. The elemental
expressions of energy are transmutations or step-downs of primary energy. They are like
the patterns or ripples generated by the primary respiratory system. Elemental energy is
expressed as five particular qualities: earth, water, fire, air and ether/space. These five qualities interweave to form energy patterns which underlie our mental, emotional and physical
states.[38] All the organs of the body can be categorized according to the predominant element
which governs their function.

Elemental energy is distributed around the body along certain channels known as *meridians*
and *nadis*. According to classical yoga theory, the body's neurological network is a correlate,
or reflection, of the underlying network of *nadis*. Dr Elmer Green of the Menninger
Foundation describes that this network consists of 'filaments of superphysical, but real, substance not yet detected by instruments'.[39] The meridian channels used in acupuncture are
believed to be significant parts of this network.

Chakras

At the places where many of these channels meet, larger gateways of energy are created.
These are the *chakras*, a Sanskrit word which literally translates as 'wheel'. There are six
(some sources describe seven) major chakras located along the midline of the body, acting as
major vortices through which subtle energy passes (see Figure 8.4).[40] Each major chakra is
externalized in the physical body in the form of nerve ganglia and plexi, and also as one of
the endocrine glands. The functioning of these organs is directly related to the balance of
energy which passes through their corresponding chakra. When all the chakras are open and
operating in balance, it indicates that the person is fully integrated in both body and mind.

Dr Viola Frymann suggests that it is possible to tune in to the motion patterns within each
chakra and thereby recognize any imbalance in their function.[41] Furthermore, she states that
the function of these vortices can be influenced towards a state of health through the use of
the physician's hands. As Dr Frymann points out, the presence of this subtle energy network
implies that,

Man is not the physical body, the emotions or the mind: these are
merely the instruments that enable him to function in the physical,
emotional and mental realms, and it behooves us to study and
understand the anatomy and physiology of these instruments if
we are to treat man as a totality[42]

She concludes,

None of these individual aspects – body, energy, emotion, or mind –
is really you, any more than you are the clothes you wear. Rather,
you are an eternal spirit and these aspects are like the garments
you put on to function in a particular area.[43]

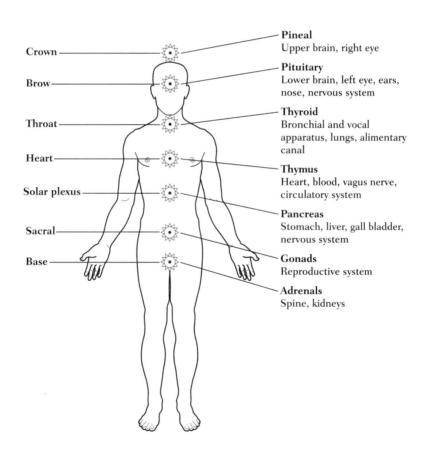

Pineal
Upper brain, right eye

Pituitary
Lower brain, left eye, ears,
nose, nervous system

Thyroid
Bronchial and vocal
apparatus, lungs, alimentary
canal

Thymus
Heart, blood, vagus nerve,
circulatory system

Pancreas
Stomach, liver, gall bladder,
nervous system

Gonads
Reproductive system

Adrenals
Spine, kidneys

Crown

Brow

Throat

Heart

Solar plexus

Sacral

Base

Figure 8.4: Major chakras

211

Staying with primary energy

The network of elemental energy distributes differentiated qualities of the Breath of Life, creating and supporting individual characteristics of mind and body. However, at their basis is the essential energy of the Breath of Life itself, organized around the midline axis of the body and expressed as rhythmic, tidal unfoldments. It is within this fundamental expression of energy that our ordering principle, the original matrix of health, is distributed. Therefore, working with primary respiratory motion has a profound influence on the entire system, and may obviate the need to work with the differentiated qualities of elemental energy distributed through the chakras or meridians.

It must be emphasized that in craniosacral work the focus of treatment is on employing the intrinsic forces of the patient's *own* primary respiratory system, and *not* in trying to channel energy from the therapist or elsewhere, as in some other forms of healing. As Dr Becker points out, 'The sole purpose is to arouse the total resources of the patient's own physiological structures.'[44]

Prevention as well as cure

The primary respiratory system brings the subtlest life breath into the body, carrying the intrinsic forces which organize the physiological functioning of our cells and tissues. This interface between essential life-energy and physical form has great significance for our health. Disturbances of function first manifest in the tidal expressions of primary respiratory motion; these disorders then act as precursors to physical illness. In other words, the primary respiratory system reflects imbalances of function before they become established as physical illness. Therefore, by working with inertial patterns within the primary respiratory system it is possible to treat problems *before* they manifest as structural and functional changes in the body.

In this way craniosacral treatment is profoundly preventative, addressing many sub-clinical states before they develop into something more severe or chronic. If a problem is dealt with at these origins of function, many other complications can be avoided. Furthermore, in situations where we 'just don't feel right' but where conventional medical tests have found nothing wrong, the causes can frequently be traced to problems of inertia within the primary respiratory system.

Establishing and maintaining a healthy and balanced expression of primary respiratory motion is at the foundation of good health. The Breath of Life is the key which can address the very core of illness.

Cutting edge

Albert Einstein once remarked, 'I didn't achieve anything through my rational mind.'[45] However, in the modern medical approach everything has to be analysed and measured with scientific apparatus, and then tested with double-blind trials in order to find acceptance. Although many of the subtle phenomena produced by the Breath of Life have yet to be proved by these methods, this doesn't mean that they do not exist. This is not a cop-out from scientific investigation but an acknowledgement that there are certain realms beyond the scope of what can currently be measured. Einstein also commented, 'The most beautiful thing we can experience is the mysterious. It is at the source of all true art and science.'[45]

Many of the functions of the Breath of Life are perhaps so close, so intrinsic that their presence often bypasses us. Nevertheless, these subtle phenomena have been experienced and tested by many practitioners working in the field, checking their results in the 'laboratory of life'. Even after more than 60 years since its development, the craniosacral concept is still at the cutting edge of a holistic understanding of how we function.

9

STRESS AND TRAUMA

The body's life is the life of sensations and emotions.
The body feels real hunger, real thirst, real joy in
the sun or snow, real pleasure in the smell of roses
or the look of a lilac bush; real anger, real sorrow,
real tenderness, real warmth, real passion, real hate,
real grief. All the emotions belong to the body and
are only recognized by the mind.

D. H. LAWRENCE

THE NATURE OF STRESS AND TRAUMA

The world breaks everyone and afterwards many are strong
in the broken places.[1]
ERNEST HEMINGWAY

Stress is a familiar experience to all of us because it is an inescapable part of life. We all know what stress feels like, whether we call it nerves, tension, frustration, worry, strain or pressure. We may recognize it when we have to meet a deadline, can't pay a bill, when we are caught in a traffic jam, or if an ill-tempered boss calls our name. The word 'stress' is used in many different ways. The *Penguin Medical Encyclopaedia* sees stress as 'any influence which disturbs the natural equilibrium of the body'.[2] Another definition of stress is 'a constraining or impelling force'.[3] We find ourselves under stress when demands are made upon us which our physiology has to respond and adapt to.

Positive stress

All change is potentially stressful, but then so are boredom and stasis. However, it's not just the stressful events themselves, but how we respond to them that determines the outcome. Stress can provide us with great benefits. Some degree of stress is necessary to motivate our enthusiasm for life and many people eagerly seek the delights and achievements of facing and mastering challenging events. In the Chinese language, the character for the word 'crisis' combines the symbols for the words 'danger' and 'opportunity'.

Through the challenges of stressful events we can grow in strength and confidence. Stress can be the spark that pushes us to progress in our chosen profession, that demands for better environmental conditions, that provides the impetus to sort out relationships and make creative changes in our lives. Stress can be seen as the irritation in the oyster that makes the pearl. Perhaps the difference between the stress of failure and frustration and other beneficial kinds of stress is in how we are able to process their forces.

Trauma

Trauma is altogether a more severe form of stress and it is always unpleasant. Although trauma is also perhaps an unavoidable part of life, it too can lead to great benefit if its effects can be resolved. Trauma may occur as a single powerful and overwhelming event or as a series of repetitive stressful experiences which accumulate. A car accident, a fall, an emotionally cold parent, a tooth extraction or a difficult birth are common examples.

How we respond to trauma is also an individual matter. It is only when our physiology becomes overwhelmed that we then suffer from longer-lasting consequences. The following pages contain a summary of the development of traumatic patterning and the principles of its treatment using craniosacral approaches. A more in-depth description of working with trauma can be found in the remarkable and insightful book *Waking the Tiger* by Dr Peter Levine.[4]

Traumatic patterning

The body's primal impulse when faced with a stressful or traumatic event is to contract. Contraction of the tissues is an integral part of our protective response. However, contractions remain in the body if the forces which caused them are unresolved. In the body's attempt to minimalize disruption, unresolved traumatic forces become focused at particular locations. Thus the imprints of trauma become centred in the form of inertial fulcrums, which organize patterns of disturbance. In this way we become patterned by traumatic experiences and by how our intrinsic health is able to accommodate for them. By addressing these physiological roots of trauma, the craniosacral practitioner is able to facilitate profound shifts in habitual patterns of distress.

Retraumatization

In the 1960s and 1970s it became popular in various therapeutic circles to encourage the expression of repressed experiences in order to 'get rid' of them. Cathartic approaches to treatment were developed in which the patient was asked to dramatize their pain or anger, hurt or terror, etc. Catharsis might also involve the body, which could be encouraged to retrace and relive its patterns of trauma and distress. However, many therapists have since found that, instead of resolving the trauma, catharsis often results in the patient becoming retraumatized. Furthermore, the re-enactment of patterns of distress would frequently further reinforce the trauma. Therefore ways of working with trauma have been developed that follow the instinctual intelligence of the body, rather than 'digging up the dirt' or using confrontation. To understand how these approaches work, an appreciation is needed about how traumatization occurs in the first place. This involves an understanding of the biological basis of trauma.

PHYSIOLOGY OF STRESS AND TRAUMA

Trauma is part of a natural physiological process that
simply has not been allowed to be completed.[5]
DR PETER LEVINE

The key to resolving trauma lies in our physiology. Imagine that you are walking through a jungle. As you are making your way along a jungle path, you think you hear a rustling in the bushes just ahead. You stop in your tracks. Your senses become heightened as you scan the bushes, listening for any more sounds. This is a state of *active alert*. If you see or hear nothing, you may then return to a state of relaxation and cheerfully continue on your way.

The fight or flight response

However, let's say that you hear some more rustling and then see something moving through the bushes. Your physiological response will stay in a state of active alert. If then a lion appears from out of the bushes and confronts you on the path ahead, what kind of body responses do you think you might feel? It's probable that your heartbeat would increase in order to pump more blood around your body, blood pressure would rise, your muscles would tense, breathing would quicken (to provide more oxygen) and your eyes may dilate. Furthermore, you might start sweating as your skin gets ready to cool down in anticipation of any over-heating produced by conflict. There would also be a tendency to turn pale as a result of blood being diverted to your muscles, your mouth might go dry as the salivary glands stop producing saliva, and other functions less important for immediate survival, such as digestion, slow down or stop altogether. Your body would move from 'active alert' to a state of *fight or flight*.[6]

The fight or flight response prioritizes the vital metabolic functions of the body. This assists us in either fighting or running away when faced with danger, by diverting the body's resources towards the most important task in hand: survival.

A successful outcome

If the lion saw you and then ran back into the bushes, within a short period of time your fight or flight response would diminish and you would return to a state of active alert. This stage would remain until you felt the danger was completely over, when you could relax again. However, if the lion didn't run away but crouched down on the path ahead, as if ready to pounce, your fight or flight response would continue. All your energies would become mobilized. Since it's probably not a good idea to try to fight a lion, you would most likely turn and run as fast as you could. Let's say you were just outside a village and you managed to make it back to a hut, get inside and slam the door behind you. Again, within a short time, the fight or flight response would diminish and you could return, first to a state of active alert, and then relaxation. The energy which became mobilized in your body would have been used to great effect. You escaped the danger. There would likely be no traumatization and you might even feel a sense of achievement and empowerment.

Shock

Let's say, however, that the lion caught up with you as you tried to run. If you became trapped, you would be unable to express the physiological energies which had mobilized in your body as part of the fight or flight response. This would lead to a trapping of these powerful forces in the body, causing a state of *shock*. Shock occurs when our responses to danger are overwhelmed.

Two of the primary elements which constitute a state of shock are *freezing* and *dissociation*. Freezing happens when we realize that we can't escape. There is nowhere left for us to run and we become immobilized. At this point, the cranial rhythmic impulse comes to a sudden halt (see Shutdown, page 224). Dr Peter Levine points out, 'As in the Greek myth of Medusa, the human confusion that may ensue when we stare death in the face can turn us to stone. We may literally freeze in fear, which will result in the creation of traumatic symptoms.'[7] Dissociation involves a splitting or separation of our consciousness from the situation, so that if we suffer injury our experience of the pain is minimalized. This is a very intelligent and useful response! A child who is helpless, for example, against a bullying teacher may react in the same way. So may a victim of violence, rape or traumatic accident.

Animal kingdom

Let's look at how the trauma response acts as a survival mechanism in the animal kingdom. In the wild, many animals of prey have learned not to eat carrion. Experience has taught them that ingesting dead meat often gives them a bad stomach, so they eat only fresh food. Therefore playing dead can be a useful strategy.

If you have ever watched a wildlife film with a cheetah chasing an antelope, you may have seen the antelope go into a state of freezing and dissociation if it becomes overpowered. From the outside it appears that the antelope is dead. The cheetah may then prod the antelope to check if it is alive and, if there is no response, may drag the antelope away to share later with its cubs.

Reassociation

However, if someone drove up in a landrover just at this time, the cheetah may run away. The antelope will start to come round in a process of *reassociation*. The energy of shock trapped in its body will begin to manifest and discharge, causing it to shake. The shaking usually begins with the antelope's legs and may spread through its whole body. It will then stand up and, after a few more shakes, make its escape. It will have re-entered a state of fight or flight. If the antelope perceives that the danger has passed, it will revert back to a state of active alert. When it feels secure that there is no more immediate threat, it can then return to relaxation. In this instance the antelope will not have become traumatized. It will have passed through a traumatic experience, but will have been able to dissipate the shock. However, a state of *traumatization* occurs if for some reason the antelope is prevented from processing the energies bound up in its body.

Social and cultural influences

It seems that we humans are not as efficient as some wild animals at processing the effects of shock. Social and cultural influences, mediated by our higher brain centres, affect the way we react. Instead of following our instinctual responses, our brain cortex may override the situation. We often become prevented from naturally discharging the physiological effects of shock, which then remain trapped inside. For example, when someone slams into the back of your car you will probably feel shaky, but instead of discharging the imploded energy of shock ... you may simply exchange insurance details.[8] If you work in an office and your boss shouts your name, you may go into a fight or flight response. However, in this instance fighting or fleeing may not be successful strategies as either will probably get you the sack! Therefore, all the energy that has become mobilized in your body has nowhere to go. Dr Peter Levine compares this to putting your foot down hard on both the accelerator and the brake at the same time.[9]

Getting overwhelmed

Essentially, the imprints of traumatic experiences become retained when our capacity to dissipate them is overwhelmed. There are tremendous forces which can be accessed when we enter a fight or flight response. Great feats of strength and endurance become possible. If all this energy is thwarted, it implodes and can remain trapped in the body. We may then lack the capacity to do anything other than contain this energy as best we can. Importantly, if our traumatic experiences are restimulated at some point in the future, unless the resources to resolve them have been developed we will simply get overwhelmed again. Often, this retraumatization occurs when we are in situations reminiscent of the original trauma.

Symptoms of trauma

The imprints of unresolved traumatic experiences may lead to a variety of clinical symptoms. Typically, at first, a traumatized person suffers from extreme sensitivity, flashbacks, hesitation, nervousness, mistrust, mood swings or panic attacks. A little later, as the tissues of the body become arranged in relationship to the presence of trauma, various other symptoms may develop, such as digestive disturbances, headaches, jaw tension, chronic fatigue, asthma, urinary problems and back pain.[10]

An accumulative process

The effects of stress and trauma can be accumulative, as new incidents become superimposed over previous ones. As the responses of inertia and dissociation require a lot of energy to maintain, the available biodynamic forces of the body can become correspondingly reduced, so diminishing our resources to deal with any new incidents. Therefore, a traumatized person tends to get more easily overwhelmed. Many researchers have noted how chronic and repetitive stress weakens the effectiveness of any future stress response.[11] As Peter Levine observes, 'When we are unable to flow through trauma and complete instinctive responses, these incompleted actions often undermine our lives.'[12]

Long-term effects

The physiological responses to stress and trauma are the same whether we are faced with a situation of real danger or only imagined danger. For example, if we are walking in the grass we may see something on the ground that looks like a snake. On taking a closer look we realize that, in fact, it's a piece of rope. Nevertheless, the same physiological responses occur. It's only when we realize that there is no danger that we relax. As long as an incident is *perceived* as being stressful, our fight or flight response is activated. If the actual or perceived stress is prolonged, then the fight or flight response continues, possibly for long periods of time.

For those people who suffer from long-term stress or traumatization, the effects on the body may be substantial. Consider what may happen physiologically over time if our fight or flight response is continually aroused. Muscular contraction will persist, blood pressure will stay high, breathing will stay rapid, digestion will be diminished and a whole host of hormonal changes, which are an integral part of the stress response, remain.[13] Sooner or later the adaptive mechanisms to prolonged stress become overwhelmed; it is then that health can start to break down. Furthermore, as this response is not under voluntary control, you can't ask someone who is faced by threat or danger (or who simply thinks that they are) to relax!

Emotional coupling

When faced with trauma, it's quite likely that emotions such as fear, rage, grief or despair may arise at the same time. If we become overwhelmed, these emotions can also get retained within any resultant inertia (see also Chapter 8, The Mind–Body Continuum, page 196). Thus, the retained imprint of trauma can include a physiological pattern which becomes coupled with an intense emotion. If the trauma is restimulated at some time in the future, it is probable there will be a rekindling of the associated fear, grief or rage.

Our responses to life thus become conditioned by our earlier traumas. Sigmund Freud recognized the biological basis of this tendency to remain conditioned. He stated that, 'After severe shock ... the dream life continually takes the patient back to the situation of his disaster from which he awakens with renewed terror ... The patient has undergone a physical fixation to the trauma.'[14] Therefore, for a resolution of these experiences to occur the message of healing has to get right into our cells.

SHUTDOWN AND DISSOCIATION

I'm not afraid of dying, I just don't want to be there when it happens.
WOODY ALLEN

Fragmentation of function

It is when our resources to respond effectively to a situation are overwhelmed that traumatization results. One of the chief characteristics of overwhelm and traumatization is the instinctual cutting off from sensations. This dissociation is a very useful short-term strategy, but perhaps not so helpful if perpetuated over time. It helps us to cope, but doesn't help in the resolution of trauma. A person who remains dissociated may appear 'spaced out', forgetful or out of touch, and cannot function with a sense of integration and flow. This frequently affects the natural midline orientation of the Breath of Life, and is clearly marked by inertia in the subtle rhythms of primary respiratory motion.

Cutting off

When dissociated we are unable to stay present with certain parts of ourselves. Thus, staying in contact with anyone else is also very difficult. It may be hard to make eye contact or we may experience difficulty being still. We may respond by filling our lives with constant activity to avoid the painful sensations inside us, or we may give up and go into 'hibernation'. To some degree we are probably all dissociated, because it is likely that we all have areas of ourselves that we do not fully inhabit.

Dissociation always involves some degree of being separated from physical sensation. When dissociated we are not fully *in* our bodies (i.e. fully incarnated) and are therefore unable to operate at our full potential. For example, we may not be able to 'find our feet' or we may live 'in our heads' or we may have 'lost heart'. While dissociation gives a certain release from pain and difficulty, it is quite different from the true freedom that results from the problem not being there. If any sensations are later triggered in an area of the body where dissociation is experienced, they may be felt as threatening or even retraumatizing.

I was treating a victim of torture who had been subjected to electric shocks and repeatedly kicked in the stomach during a long imprisonment. He was left with a hollow and numb feeling in his abdomen. This feeling of numbness was his way of cutting off from the sensations of his painful experience. However, he was consequently left with digestive problems, headaches and depression. A woman with a back injury described how she had been 'knocked sideways' when her car was hit by another driver, and that she had been feeling 'out of sorts' ever since. Her dissociation was created as she became literally pushed out to one side from the traumatic force of the accident.

Denial

A degree of unconscious denial is always present with dissociation. Usually, the part of the person that is dissociated doesn't know that it is. If you ask them how they feel, they will probably tell you (often in a higher-pitched voice than their normal tone) that they are 'fine'. They may even say that they've never felt better! This is because the body secretes large amounts of adrenaline and endorphins (natural opiates) when traumatized, which can create feelings of euphoria. In the course of treating a few religious fanatics, I've noticed how they sometimes come under this category. It seems that although some people may describe euphoric and 'cosmic' experiences, they actually seem to be deeply traumatized and out of touch with their body. In the same way, a victim of a stabbing or shooting may be unaware of their injury until they see blood coming from their wound. There are many stories of soldiers at war who have had this experience.

A common experience

Traumatization is actually a common experience, often arising from events that are widely accepted as 'normal'. It may have occurred as a result of a difficult birth, emotional neglect or surgery. One young girl I was treating had nightmares for months after feeling traumatized from an appendix operation. An 82-year-old retired doctor came for treatment because he was experiencing a great and overwhelming feeling of fear. In a recurring dream, this fear came to him in the vision of an icy, cold woman who put an injection into his spine which took away his sense of power. Interestingly, he revealed that some 50 years earlier a nurse had performed a lumbar puncture to remove some of his cerebrospinal fluid for medical tests. Anaesthetic drugs do not detract from the traumatic impact of surgery, they just numb the effects (as well as increasing the level of toxicity in the body). For these reasons, although surgery is often a necessary intervention, Dr Becker refers to it as 'organized trauma'.[15]

Perpetuation and re-enactment

Old traumas often get perpetuated or even reinforced in the course of our lives. We seem to have a remarkable and mysterious capacity for attracting experiences which resonate with previous ones. A woman who was physically abused as a child may marry a violent abuser. The violent abuser himself was probably a victim of abuse ... and so it goes. How often is it that acts of violence are perpetrated by victims of violence?

Sometimes it seems that traumas repeat themselves as part of an attempt to seek their resolution. I was working with a patient who suffered from frequent low back pain. During one of her sessions she moved into a curled-up position and started to shake. She shared afterwards that she was born in a breech position (bottom first) and life had been 'a bumpy ride' ever since. That same evening after the treatment she fell bottom first down a long flight of stairs. Thankfully she was able to access the resources to work through the effects of her traumatization.

Shutdown

In craniosacral work the practitioner has a clear and direct handle into the effects of trauma. Whenever states of overwhelm and freezing are experienced, there is a sudden cessation of the cranial rhythmic impulse, called a *shutdown*. This is a palpable phenomenon, which is felt by the practitioner as the cranial rhythmic impulse coming to an abrupt stop. Shutdowns occur due to the presence of unresolved shock held in the system, often appearing when a traumatic memory is contacted. A shutdown is a protective response which involves an instinctive contraction from life. It usually lasts anything from a few seconds to a few minutes. However, where a person's resources have become more severely overwhelmed it can continue for even longer. In a shutdown the tissues are less able to take up the potency of the Breath of Life. This leads to a disconnection from their original matrix of health.

A physiological stop sign

When a shutdown appears during treatment, it can be viewed as a kind of physiological stop sign which needs to be honoured. It's actually not possible for trauma to be resolved while still in a shutdown. This is because the Breath of Life can't be expressed and some degree of dissociation is always present. As with any kind of problem, it cannot be worked with if we are not actually there! Furthermore, issues of trauma can only truly be healed when a relationship to them is found from a place of health, rather than from a place of overwhelm.

The cranial rhythmic impulse only starts up again from a shutdown when the resources that enable us to stay present can be built up or contacted. When the cranial rhythmic impulse resumes, it indicates that the process of working through a trauma can then continue. In the mean time, confronting someone in a shutdown will probably further overwhelm their resources. The presence of resources are critical if overwhelm is to be avoided.

RESOURCES

Believing that a loving, intelligent Maker of man had deposited in his
body in some place or throughout the whole system drugs in abundance to
cure all infirmities, on every voyage of exploration I have been able to

bring back a cargo of indisputable truths, that all the remedies necessary
to health exist in the human body.[16]
DR A. T. STILL

In situations where patients are in states of overwhelm, the priority of craniosacral treatment is to help build and develop their resources. These resources can then provide a solid foundation for the resolution of traumatic forces and the consequent expression of health.

A resource is anything that helps to support health and balance. A good experience can be resource, as can a place or an inner capacity from which we draw support. Resources create physiological responses in the body. When a resource is contacted we may feel sensations of reconnection, settling, expansion or lightness. Resources help us to stay present and give the capacity to relate to traumatization without getting overwhelmed.

Inner and outer resources

We may find resources in many aspects of our lives. Resources can be physical, emotional, psychological, spiritual or environmental. They often derive from an activity that we do, such as exercise, dance or a hobby. Environmental resources may include a place where we can go to recharge, a supportive friend, a pet or a piece of music that inspires us. These can help to access or build up inner resources. Inner resources may include places in our bodies that feel OK, a happy memory, trust, wisdom, experience, a sense of our own strength, instinctual responses and, of course, the Breath of Life. Dissociation can also be seen as a kind of resource because it provides relative comfort, helping us to cope if overwhelmed. Other resources include things like family, home, laughter, meditation, favourite clothes, a piece of jewellery, good food, touch, books, therapy, trees and space. Resources are very specific to each individual.

One man diagnosed with terminal cancer was told that he had only a short time to live. After hearing this he decided to stop work and spend the rest of his days following whatever made him happy. He went to his local video store and bought copies of his favourite Marx Brothers films. These films had always been one of his greatest resources. He thought that if he were going to die soon, he might as well die laughing. Over the next weeks he sat in front of his television set immersed in laughter. When he returned to his doctor a couple of months later, all signs of his cancer had disappeared.[17]

Social support

There can be no doubt that positive social support is an important resource for the prevention and cure of many diseases. A study carried out at Stanford University by psychiatrist Dr David Spiegel in the mid-1970s points to this fact.[18] Dr Spiegel led support groups for women with advanced cancer. His intent was to provide a support system for women in which they were able to talk about their day-to-day problems. He aimed to show how this would improve the quality of their lives. To Dr Spiegel's surprise, when he went back to check on these women a decade later, long after the support groups had disbanded, he found that the women in these groups survived twice as long as others. They lived an average of 18 months longer than women who did not have the same support. This is much longer than any cancer medications could provide.

Bali cow

In modern society, despite the many benefits provided by technological advancement, many people experience isolation, alienation and a lack of social support. The great difference between the way our modern world and some traditional cultures deal with problems was graphically illustrated to me when I was staying on the Indonesian island of Bali.

I was lying on a beach (resourcing!) when a procession of local villagers started to make their way along the sand. They were singing and banging drums whilst leading a cow down to the water's edge. They steered the cow right into the water, splashing the frightened animal as they whistled and shouted at the top of their voices. I asked one of the villagers what was going on. He explained that a young man from their village had been deluded into thinking that the cow was a beautiful woman, and had consequently been discovered making love to the cow. The villagers' ritual was to help break the spell of this terrible delusion, so that the youth could be freed from his ignorance and suffering. The whole community had come out to lend their assistance and support.

I was deeply struck by the fact that this problem, which would no doubt be hidden by shame and guilt in the West, involved the boy's whole family and the rest of the village. There seemed to be no blame, and each member of the community felt a responsibility to act in a positive way to help heal the situation.

Identification

The process of healing is never just about identifying problems, but involves accessing the resources that can help resolve these problems. No matter how much traumatization has occurred, the reality is that we are never just our pattern of trauma. We are more than just our experiences; there is always the *being* who is having the experiences. However, we can often get stuck in an experience, particularly if it is overwhelming. When this happens, the trauma pattern becomes a major fulcrum with which we identify and which shapes our lives. We may even join a support group with other victims of a similar experience. While this may prove valuable, our identification with the trauma can sometimes remain strong.

Consider for a moment, with what do you identify in your life? Are you able to identify with your health?

A resourcing exercise (1)

Take a minute or two to consider the resources you have in your life. Close your eyes and bring an image of a resource into your mind. What supports you? It may be a place you have been or an experience you have had. It's probably not a good idea to use the image of a person for this purpose, because this can sometimes create ambiguous feelings. Try to find a resource that is entirely supportive. Imagine yourself in a place that resources you, or with your favourite object, or recall an experience that made you feel good.

As you picture this resource, what sensations do you feel in your body?

Parasympathetic response

The involuntary part of our nervous system directs functions of the body not normally under conscious control; for example, digestion, respiration, temperature and circulation. The involuntary nervous system has two branches which operate in a reciprocal and harmonic relationship. These are called the *parasympathetic* and *sympathetic* nervous systems.

Resources tend to activate the parasympathetic nervous system. This branch is concerned with our relaxation response and mainly operates when we are in states of rest. Under its influence the physiological systems of the body, such as heartbeat and breathing, slow down and find a point of ease. However, the sympathetic nervous system is concerned with mobi-lizing the activities of the body required to deal with stress. Therefore, threat or danger activates the sympathetic branch. The fight or flight response is mediated via the sympathetic nervous system.

The parasympathetic and sympathetic nervous systems alternate in their function. The degree to which the sympathetic branch is activated, is the degree to which the parasympathetic system cannot function. Ideally we should be able to move smoothly between both parasympathetic and sympathetic responses. However, according to Dr James Jealous, 80 per cent or more of disease is directly related to an imbalance in this interchange.[19] As resources tend to encourage a parasympathetic response, they can be used as a tool for balancing any excessive sympathetic activation. The encouragement of stillpoints of the cranial rhythmic impulse has proven very valuable in this regard.

A healing fulcrum

Whatever our resources are, they can help us to form a healthier connection to patterns of trauma. They establish a place of health from which we can then move forward with a sense of refuge and balance. They provide a kind of *healing fulcrum*. If resourced, a trauma can be revisited without getting retraumatized, enabling the pattern to be processed and discharged.

Our most fundamental resources are those which can be found within. In the craniosacral concept, the Breath of Life is considered to be an intrinsic unwavering ordering principle which regulates the physiological functions of the body, and brings integration to body and mind. When the expression of the Breath of Life is restored in places of inertia, the re-emergence of our original matrix of health takes place. If this resource can be facilitated in patterns of trauma, their dissipation results.

SHOCK AND TRAUMA SKILLS

Patients and their problems do not retrace steps to return to health.
Health is NOW.[20]
DR ROLLIN BECKER D.O.

Role of the nervous system

Traumatization remains as long as we are unable to access the resources to complete the process of its discharge. Essentially, it is not a memory of the past, but an experience carried in the present. Traumatic experiences which have not yet reached a satisfactory point of completion and resolution become perpetuated as a physiological pattern. It seems that much of the unresolved energy of a traumatized person ends up being trapped in their nervous system.

It has been found that the mid-brain and brain stem control many of the physiological responses to stress and trauma. These regions of the brain contain nerve nuclei and other nerve centres which become facilitated (i.e. irritated) in perpetuated states of overwhelm. The nervous system of a traumatized person may then feel 'wired', as it becomes held in a state of constant arousal, yet at the same time this energy may not have anywhere to go. These effects of traumatization can be palpable as a loss of primary respiratory motion in these vital centres. Instead of being able to express its natural motility in cycles of inhalation and exhalation, this area of the central nervous system becomes inertial.

Physiological switches

Through understanding the importance of primary respiratory motion to the functioning of the brain, craniosacral work can access the very origins of patterns of traumatization. Where particular 'trauma switches' in the brain centres are still turned on, they can be encouraged to dissipate their energy and return to an expression of normal primary respiratory motion. During this process of resolution, tremors and vibratory motions in the central nervous system and the fluids of the body are often palpated. This is an indication that the forces of trauma trapped in the nervous system are starting to discharge.

In the present

It has been a common misconception that past traumas need to be re-experienced in order to break the fetters of their control. This notion suggests that it is only through regression that the roots of trauma can be cut.[21] However, the reliving of a trauma pattern, by itself, does not significantly help with its resolution. It seems, more often than not, that if memories of past traumas are dredged up they simply become reactivated or even endorsed.[22,23,24] As the Dalai Lama commented during a recent talk, 'The more you indulge in thoughts or emotions, the stronger they can become.'[25] A trauma is only resolved when the forces which organize it are able to shift. To emphasize this necessitates the presence of resources.

Traumas can also only be effectively healed *in the present*, for it is here that they are held. Furthermore, our resources of health are found only in the present. Therefore, the ability to stay in touch with the present is one of the keys to trauma resolution.

Acting it out

There is certainly a usefulness in recognizing and identifying patterns of distress in order to be able to work with them. This may sometimes involve re-experiencing the sensations and feelings associated with a trauma. However, it is not the *expression* of these patterns that creates the cure. Acting out a trauma pattern to try to get rid of it may help to let off steam from the 'pressure cooker', but it doesn't necessarily mean that the heat has been turned off. If resources are not developed, and a trauma is re-experienced, it will quite likely send someone back into a state of deeper traumatization.

Completion

Nevertheless, old patterns which contain the imprints of trauma may naturally come to the surface as they begin their process of completion. When this occurs there may be an exacerbation of existing symptoms or re-experiencing of old ones, sometimes described as a 'healing crisis' (see Chapter 7). For example, feelings of pain, fear, anger or despair may surface as the trapped traumatic forces are in the process of resolving. In order to allow this resolution to complete, these experiences are best neither encouraged nor discouraged, but simply accepted as part of the healing process.

Ground rules

There are certain ground rules which can enable the safe and successful resolution of the often powerful forces involved in trauma patterns. These principles can be broadly categorized as:

- waiting at shutdowns
- building resources
- contacting resources
- staying with body sensations
- being present
- slowing things down

- having a sense of space
- facilitating the discharge of shock.

☐ *Waiting at shutdowns*

While we don't have to relive our traumas in order to find healing, we may, however, need to find a relationship to them. This relationship is not possible to establish when in a disconnected state of overwhelm and dissociation. If overwhelm is present it is indicated by the cardinal sign of a shutdown of the cranial rhythmic impulse. This wisdom of the body is important to accept. When a shutdown occurs, the priority of the practitioner is to help to build resources in the patient (see below) and wait with patience until motion resumes.

☐ *Building resources*

The building of sufficient resources is fundamental to the process of trauma resolution. This is because traumatization only occurred in the first place because resources were overwhelmed. If they are not present when a trauma is revisited, retraumatization will result. However, if resources are low, they can be developed and strengthened. This may involve a holistic health-building approach, including the establishment of a balanced lifestyle, suitable diet and adequate rest. The principal approach of building resources in craniosacral work is by the facilitation of stillpoints (see Chapter 7, Stillpoints, page 175). Stillpoints strengthen the vital reserves of the body by recharging the 'battery fluid' (cerebrospinal fluid) with potency. More resources then become available to help with the dissipation of the trauma.

☐ *Contacting resources*

In many instances we may already have sufficient resources, but just be unable to access them. There are a number of approaches which are used to help contact existing resources. The biodynamic potency carried in the fluids of the body are our primary resource for health. However, much of this potency can get bound up in inertial fulcrums, which makes it unavailable for other uses. Therefore, by resolving inertial patterns, this potency is freed up and our available resources are strengthened. Furthermore, if we are able to tune in to and connect with the long tide or mid-tide operating beneath a pattern of trauma, it can help our physiology to resonate and align with these deeper expressions of health.

Whether we find resources in an internal capacity, an object, an experience or a sensation, we can draw on their aid in times of need. No matter how bad things get, there is nearly always something somewhere that feels OK for us. This feeling of OK-ness may be experienced when recalling a pleasant memory or a place in the body where we can contact good sensations.

A resourcing exercise (2)

One way to connect with existing resources is to bring your attention into your body and see if you can find a place where you feel good sensations. Even if this place is just the tip of your little finger or toe, you will probably be able to find somewhere that feels OK! Having established this connection, you can then begin to explore the places in your body where you feel some difficulty or painful sensations.

Sit quietly in a chair and take a couple of minutes to bring your attention to the sensations that you feel in your body. You may want to start at your feet and then work your way up, scanning the body for sensations as you go along. Begin to notice the places where you feel discomfort and other places where you feel good sensations. Just be open to whatever you feel. Try to accept whatever is there without making any interpretations or judgements.

Select a place in your body where you feel some good sensations. Take a couple of minutes to let your attention rest there. What do you notice? Take a few deep breaths into this place and enjoy the sensations that you feel. When you have established a good connection with these sensations, gently bring your attention to a place or an area of your body where you feel a pain or some other difficulty. What sensations do you notice there? See if you can stay there for a short time (but take care not to get overwhelmed). If you feel that things are getting too difficult, then bring your attention back to the place in your body where you feel OK.

After a minute or so of staying with the difficulty, again bring your attention back to the place where you feel good sensations. Take a little more time to resource in this place. Then, again bring your attention back to the place of difficulty. What do you notice? Move back and forth a few times between your sensations of difficulty and a place of resource. Do you notice any changes taking place?

The purpose of this exercise is to help establish a place in the body where we can go to resource. It may then be possible to relate to a trauma pattern without getting overwhelmed. However, if you do feel overwhelmed or uncomfortable at any stage of this process, then just stop doing it. If this is your experience, you may wish to seek the help of a qualified practitioner to help you through.

☐ *Staying with body sensations*

Tracking the sensations in the body can help us to stay in touch with a difficult experience and prevent dissociation. Staying with sensations involves a deep trust in our instinctive responses and a sufficient feeling of safety and containment to be able to follow them. Someone who is severely dissociated, however, may find this hard to carry out. That's fine, for dissociation is an intelligent response that may need to be explored before the person is ready to come back into their body.

Staying in touch with sensations can be cultivated by developing what Professor Eugine Gendlin (the developer of 'Focusing') calls our 'felt sense'.[26] This is the bodily sense of how we experience something. It is a general feeling which may be composed of physical sensations, emotional tones and perhaps also images. Franklyn Sills describes it as an inner realm 'which allows access to how we hold meaning in an embodied way'.[27]

As long as we are in touch with our felt sense, the process of transforming traumatic symptoms can naturally progress. If we dissociate, we can try to gently reconnect with our felt sense once again. This process of reassociation helps the resolution of trauma to continue and complete. In this regard, Dr Peter Levine affirms that, 'Body sensation, rather than intense emotion, is the key to healing trauma.'[28]

Reassociating

A patient who had fallen seven feet from a ladder, and injured his shoulder and back in the process, started to experience a trembling in his body during a craniosacral treatment. This trembling was noticeable, first in his solar plexus, but soon spread to his legs. However, he found it difficult to stay with these sensations as it brought up a lot of anxiety for him. He reached a point when he went into a shutdown and seemed to 'disappear'. I asked him, 'Where are you just now?' He replied, 'I feel like I'm floating somewhere up by the ceiling!' I asked, 'How do you feel up there?' 'It feels quite nice!', was the reply. I suggested that he should stay there for as long as he needed, but also reassured him that his shaking was just a natural process of shock discharging from his nervous system. Even though he was dissociated, he was quite present with this fact. After a few minutes he started to feel ready to come back into his body. He was able to take a few deep breaths and begin to notice the sensations of trembling in his legs once more. Little by little, as he felt sufficiently resourced, he was able to allow these sensations to move through him in intermittent cycles. As he did this, the shaking was able to complete. Once the shock had discharged from his system, it didn't take long for his back and shoulder symptoms to improve.

☐ *Being present*

The ability to be in the present seems vital for the process of trauma healing. It can be important for the patient to recognize that although a trauma may be restimulated, it's usually not the case that real danger exists in the present time. However, when a trauma pattern is encountered, because of the difficult sensations that are evoked there may be a tendency to lose sense of where we are by either 'spacing out' or spinning into the vortex of trauma. Being present involves being in touch with our sensations and having a sense of where we are with things. As we noted, it is only in the present that our health exists, and therefore where healing can occur.

For example, during a craniosacral therapy session, a patient of mine had the presence to recognize that she was feeling terror when she recalled the image of her abusing step-father entering her room. In this recognition she was able to be *with* her terror rather than *becoming* it. She was able to stay with the sensations she felt in her body without becoming consumed by them or dissociating. As the sensations of terror, then disgust, anger and finally strength moved through her, she was able to stay present with them, until the process of resolution was completed.

When present, it is possible to work with the delicate balance of staying with our sensations and not getting overwhelmed. The quality of a practitioner's presence can be a valuable support for this balance, helping to provide containment and safety for the patient's experience.

☐ *Slowing things down*

When trauma patterns are restimulated, the sensations, feelings and images which arise are usually very powerful, and may easily again become overwhelming. Like a dam ready to burst, there is a tendency for too much to happen too quickly and for a person to slip into states of hyperarousal. However, if the sluices of a dam are opened slowly, the water can then flow out without any problem.

When a trauma is re-experienced, a process of slow renegotiation needs to occur to prevent overwhelm from occurring again.[29] This renegotiation involves moving back into relationship with the trauma in small and manageable portions. If we are able to take things slowly, we will be able to process even substantial degrees of traumatization ... bit by bit, in a progressive way. As hyperarousal states are usually marked by rapid and shallow breathing, taking some slow and deep breaths is an effective way to slow down the process. This can help to prevent spinning out of control in a dissociated state.

☐ *Having a sense of space*

A sense of space is also needed in order to find a relationship to trauma so that the patient can work with it, rather than 'becoming' it. This can obviate any tendency to get sucked into a cycle of retraumatization and overwhelm. Therefore, when a trauma pattern is accessed it's helpful to stay on the edge of it, rather than diving in. From the edge, it's then possible to work with a little at a time. As this is done, the edge can move and a little more can be worked with.

Accessing a place inside from where we can *observe* our sensations, without getting too drawn into them, enables us to witness any arising experiences with a sense of space. This inner 'witness' is not an emotion or an attitude, but a state of awareness which can register sensations and emotions impartially and without judgement. Developing an inner witness can help the patient to relate to powerful forces which would otherwise be overwhelming.

☐ *Facilitating the discharge of shock*

The imploded energies associated with traumatization can be considerable. Nevertheless they may be transformed safely and effectively simply by following the wisdom in the body and its needs. When the conditions are ripe, our instinctual responses – which may have become thwarted and overwhelmed – are able to move towards a point of completion. This involves the discharge of any held-in shock.

When shock discharges from the body, it tends to come out in the form of trembling, twitching or shaking. Typically, this trembling can be palpated by practitioners in the motion of the patient's cerebrospinal fluid and central nervous system. Larger movements may then start, often in the limbs, and perhaps spread through the whole body. This shaking is a sign that the body is dissipating its held-in shock. While this is happening, tissue memories may also come to the surface. Simply allowing this process will enable it to complete.

When we are able to move through trauma, we may rightly feel a sense of achievement. We will perhaps have stared death in the face, confronted our deepest fears, and discovered our own instinctual abilities and sense of power in the process. We may then be in a position to change our habitual and conditioned responses, and find new ways to meet life's demands. Moreover, because each one of us has probably experienced traumatization, it is a journey to wholeness in which we all can participate.

10

PREGNANCY, BIRTH AND CHILDREN

Ships go East and ships go West

Blown by the self-same gale

It is not the gale, but the set of the sail

That directs the way they shall go.[1]

ELLA WHEELER WILCOX

START OF LIFE

The Breath of Life inspires
The eternal womb of the
Divine Mother
Who conceives and gives birth
to the promise of God in every being.
Thus our well is eternal
The Breath of Life fills us
Again and again.[2]
HAVEN TREVINO

Effects of birth

The birth process is one of the most formative events of our lives. We have to undergo considerable forces of compression in the journey through our mother's pelvis to be born. This can have a great impact on the functioning of the primary respiratory mechanism, and may create patterning that remains with us into adulthood. If you consider a young tree which grows with a prevailing wind blowing on one side, the whole tree will become inclined in that direction. The same thing happens in the human body. If we undergo stresses and strains during our birth which are not resolved, our whole structure organizes in relationship to the influence which they exert.[3]

The retention of stresses and strains introduced during the birth process is a frequent occurrence. When leading cranial osteopath Dr Viola Frymann conducted research in San Diego, she found that 88 per cent of the 1,250 babies who were examined showed evidence of birth trauma.[4]

Early consciousness

Historically, there has been a common belief that somehow babies are incapable of registering or remembering their feelings. Even up until the early part of the 20th century, surgery was frequently carried out on babies without the use of anaesthetic drugs and, in some places, procedures such as circumcision are still performed in this way. However, anyone who has had the opportunity to observe how a baby responds to its experiences will understand just how sensitive he or she actually is. As obstetrician Dr Frederick Leboyer points out, 'Blindly, madly, we assume that the newborn baby feels nothing. In fact, he feels ...

237

everything. Everything, totally, completely, utterly, and with a sensitivity we can't even begin to imagine.'[5]

Furthermore, there is now a growing acknowledgement that even a tiny ball of developing cells soon after conception possesses the faculty of consciousness. At this very early stage, these cells can be seen to contract in response to life events – and it may be that consciousness starts even before this. A remarkable degree of primordial awareness is indicated by the numerous accounts of people who have been able to recall accurately memories of their conception under hypnosis.[6] In craniosacral work too, there are many instances of patient's accessing memories of early embryological experiences.[7] There can be little doubt that the developing embryo and foetus is a delicate and responsive being who is acutely aware of the nature and quality of its circumstances.

PRE-BIRTH

Home is the place from which I have come and to which I return.
Home is where I always am. All circumstances call me to new steps
in the dance. All sickness points me there. All sickness is
homesickness. All healing is homecoming.[8]
DIANNE M. CONNELLY

Resourcing

Before we move further into looking at how early experiences can have an impact on our lives, it's worth noting how easily this subject can restimulate any of our own patterns of trauma. Over the years of working with and teaching this subject, it has become apparent that even just talking about early trauma can bring up feelings and sensations that relate to our own situation.

As we go through some of the different issues that can arise, take a little time to notice the sensations in your own body. If you start to feel agitated, it may be that you are resonating with something being discussed. You may then wish to take a little break or do a short exercise to find a resource, such as closing your eyes and connecting with a good sensation in your body (see Chapter 9, A resourcing exercise (2), page 233). Then take a few minutes to resource yourself.

An orientating exercise

Another exercise which may be helpful if you start to feel unsteady is a practice of orientation.

Sit comfortably with your back supported. Settle into this position. Your eyes can remain either open or closed. See if you can get a sense of your midline—an imaginary line running from top to bottom through the centre of your body. Then bring your attention to your front and remind yourself that this is your front! Feel the back part of your body and be with your awareness that this is your back! Then feel the top part of your head, followed by your feet. Feel your left side, followed by your right side. Finally, bring your attention to the inside of your body and then to the outside. Again repeat the sequence, pausing for just a few seconds at each place so that you can re-orientate to each direction: midline, front–back, top–bottom, left–right, inside–outside.

You can use this exercise as frequently as you like. When you get used to it, it only takes a minute.

Stages of patterning

In psychotherapy it has long been acknowledged that our early life experiences have a major impact on our later emotional development. Many psychologists are now also realizing that the time prior to birth is also of great importance.[9,10,11,12] Dr William Emerson, one of the world's authorities on pre-natal trauma, has identified key experiences which go right back to the very beginning of our lives and which influence the patterning of both mind and body.

Expanding on the previous theory that it is our first few years which are the most formative, he takes this idea back to the time of our conception. The period from conception to birth has been named the time of *primary patterning*.[13] It is here that the foundations are set for the way in which we develop and function. Experiences during this period serve as a core layer of conditioning.

Secondary patterning is what happens from the time of birth to about the age of five.

Finally, *tertiary patterning* is what happens from the age of five onwards. As our physiological and psychological tendencies become organized during the period of primary patterning, any later patterning can be seen as mainly an 'overlay' or reaction to this.[14]

The roots of experience

The very roots of any conditioning that influences the way we function can frequently be found in early experiences. As most of our physiological and psychological patterning has been completed by the time we are able to speak, the memories of these experiences cannot be accessed through words, but in the language of the body and its sensations. Even though thoughts and feelings may become associated with the pattern, these experiences are primarily remembered in our tissues. Therefore, the tools for the resolution of these patterns can be found in our physiology rather than in our psychology.

Some of the common issues that arise during pregnancy are considered below.

Effects of trauma

The first eight weeks after conception, called the *embryonic period*, is a time of rapid development in the womb. By the end of this period, all the body's organs and systems have already formed. The remainder of pregnancy, the *foetal period*, is then concerned with the growth and refinement of these systems. Dr Emerson's clinical research indicates that any traumas which occur during pregnancy affect the particular organ or body system in the phase of most rapid progression at the time.[15]

For example, there is some evidence to suggest that heart problems can originate from a trauma suffered during the third week of pregnancy. The baby's heart begins to function at this time.[16] A condition which affects the immune system, called Systemic Lupus Erythmetosus (SLE), may similarly originate from a trauma suffered during the fourth month of pregnancy.[17] The more severe conditions, such as malformations, are often due to problems that arise during the embryonic period which affect the actual formation of the embryo's tissues. Dr John Upledger observes,

> *If something goes wrong during the first eight weeks, it may result in a*
> *defectively designed structure or system whereas, if the problem occurs*
> *after the eighth week of gestation, it will more likely result in a failure of*
> *growth, development or refinement of the involved structure or system.*[18]

The development of these later problems are usually more amenable to craniosacral treatment.

Life statements

Any traumas that the mother experiences during pregnancy, such as a fall, a car accident, emotional stress or toxicity can also be experienced by the developing baby. As a result, the baby may experience pregnancy as a time of danger and uncertainty, particularly if it undergoes traumas which relate to its very survival. Contractile responses may consequently form within the tissues of the baby and lead to patterns of inertia. These critical experiences sow the seeds for the way in which its mind and body then becomes set in later life. This can lead to the formation of important *life statements*.

A life statement is a core belief that we have about ourselves and the world. Common life statements which originate from this time are 'Life is always a struggle!' or 'Nobody loves me!' or 'The world is full of danger!' These beliefs may remain throughout life, influencing the way in which we function in all our interactions and relationships.

Implantation

Each stage of early development can carry potential risks and challenges. The implantation of the embryo into the wall of its mother's womb is one such significant event. Some estimates suggest that about 80 per cent of pregnancies do not survive implantation (often without the knowledge of the mother). If there are difficulties with implantation, it may create a traumatic response within the first cells of the developing embryo. This may lead to a patterning in its tissues, which could become associated with a life statement such as 'I can't find anything to connect to!' or 'I don't know where I belong!' or 'I'm afraid of death!' It has been found that the cells which actually implant into the mother's womb eventually migrate to form tissues around the brow of the head.[19] It may seem extraordinary, but these kinds of life statements associated with experiences of implantation often arise during craniosacral treatment of this area.

Developmental problems

A remarkable degree of organization takes place with great rapidity during the early stages of pregnancy. The central nervous system of the embryo starts to form about two weeks after conception, and the reciprocal tension membrane system, including the spinal dura, forms during the first three weeks. During the fourth week after conception the rudimentary brain is completed and the spinal column as well as the spinal cord is properly formed.[20] If trauma is experienced at this early stage it can have an impact on the functioning of these tissues. It seems feasible that a distortion in the growth centres of the spinal column may be responsible for some types of abnormal spinal curvatures in later life.[21] Furthermore, defects in the spinal cord and spina bifida can result from a complication in the development of the neural tube.[22] Other conditions such as the formation of a harelip results when something affects the fusion of the lips during the seventh week of pregnancy, and a cleft palate can result from problems with the fusion of the hard palate during the eighth to ninth week.

Responsive to stress

As well as being affected by traumatic events, a developing baby is also very sensitive to the feelings of its parents. These feelings may determine how a baby experiences the process of entering the world. Typically, factors such as whether the father is present and supportive, if there are arguments or conflicts, or stresses to do with money, home, work, or a bereavement, can have an impact. The mother's level of anxiety may resonate with echoes from her own experience of being born, or from issues such as whether she has a planned pregnancy.

If the baby is not accepted or wanted, this experience may become coupled together with any inertial patterns that are organized in its tissues. Deep-seated physical and psychological patterns about rejection may then develop, leading to life statements such as, 'Nobody cares for me' or 'I'm not wanted in this world.' On the other hand, if the baby is very much wanted the parents may have anxieties about losing it, particularly if there have been difficulties with conceiving or previous miscarriages. This can also create anxiety in the baby.

By the sixth month of pregnancy, a developing baby can begin to hear the sounds around it. Its parents' voices then serve as a reassuring and comforting influence or, if stressed, be a source of apprehension or alarm. The degree to which babies respond to the sound of their parents' voices is indicated by research into language development. This research shows that if parents talk to infants while they are still in the womb, they learn how to speak much more quickly.[23]

Sympathetic tone

The tone of a baby's muscular system becomes set according to the nature of its environment. If its mother's life circumstances cause her to be anxious or stressed, she secretes higher than normal levels of adrenaline. This passes into the bloodstream of the foetus, causing the rate of its muscle contractions to rise.[24] Therefore, the muscular activity of a baby increases if its mother is stressed. Furthermore, this increase in activity continues long after the mother's own adrenaline levels have subsided.[25]

The hormone adrenaline helps to initiate the 'fight or flight' response by increasing the activity of the sympathetic nervous system. If high levels of adrenaline persist, the tone of the baby's sympathetic nervous system becomes set at a point of greater excitability. This produces a sustained 'fight or flight' response in the baby. The increase in sympathetic nervous system activity may mean that the baby has less leeway to deal with any new stresses that it encounters. Conditions such as oversensitivity, hyperactivity, irritability and perhaps asthma or migraines can be the result.

Catherine's story

At this point, I would like to relate an incident that occurred during a craniosacral treatment with a 42-year-old woman called Catherine. Catherine was in good physical health apart from a slight tendency to asthma. However, she had frequent bouts of anxiety and found it difficult to form close relationships with men for fear that they would leave her. When I placed my hands on her frontal bone, I started to feel a pull being exerted from the reciprocal tension membranes underneath. Catherine described that she felt a peculiar and yet familiar sensation of cold down the right side of her body. As this feeling became more obvious she began to feel as if her whole body was being pulled downwards from the inside.

As she tracked these sensations in her body, Catherine started to cry. I gave her the space to let these sensations and feelings just wave through her. When, after a few minutes, I asked her what she was noticing, she could only answer, 'There's something missing down my right side!' She didn't understand this feeling or why it was there, but felt safe enough to allow herself to go deeper into it.

Again she exclaimed, 'There's something missing!', followed by more tears and shuddering movements of her body. Next she cried out, 'Where have you gone? ... Why have you left me?' She kept repeating these questions, over and over again. Her despair intensified and she then started to get overwhelmed. I encouraged her to take a few deep, slow breaths and to find a place of resource in her body. Her next statement was an emphatic cry, 'He's gone!' This was again followed by sobbing and repeated calls of, 'Where have you gone? ... Why have you left me?'

Catherine had the image that she had been a twin and that her brother had been miscarried during the early stages of pregnancy (it seems that this is a common occurence). She had consequently been left on her own. With this image in mind she entered a phase of grieving and gentle sobbing. After letting herself acknowledge all these feelings that welled up from inside of her, Catherine then felt ready to accept that her brother had died. With this acceptance she was able to lovingly say goodbye to him.

Catherine shared with me that throughout her life she had had strong feelings that something was missing, which she associated with the cold sensations down the right side of her body. Naturally, any original trauma occurred before Catherine could talk or understand what was happening. However, perhaps the memory was still being carried in her body. Whether the miscarriage of her brother actually took place or not, at the very least this experience was real for her. More significantly, after this session there was a dramatic improvement in Catherine's asthma, she no longer experienced the cold sensations down her right side, and it marked a turning point, after which she started to grow enormously in self-confidence.

Size and position of baby

If a baby grows to a large size in the womb, or if its mother's pelvis is small, the baby may find a shortage of space. This is often the case where there are twins (or more!). Any cramping within the pelvis can cause the baby to grow in an asymmetrical pattern, perhaps leading to a contraction of one side of its head or body. Something similar can also occur if the baby is in a breech position. In this case, the baby's head may be pushed up against its mother's ribs, and its arms and legs twisted.[26] These patterns may remain after birth, but are usually quite amenable to craniosacral treatment.

Umbilical insufficiency

A developing baby needs to receive a constant and well-balanced supply of nutrition for its healthy growth and development. The umbilical cord is the lifeline in the womb through which it receives food and gets rid of wastes. The umbilical cord becomes attached to the mother's placenta, which is fully formed by the third month of pregnancy. This tissue is richly supplied with blood in order to provide nutrition to the baby. The placenta also helps to filter out harmful substances so that they don't enter the baby's bloodstream. Nevertheless, some types of toxin are able to pass through.

Nutritional deficiencies in the baby can occur from a variety of causes. Naturally, it is important that a mother-to-be eats a wholesome and nutritionally balanced diet. In particular, mothers who conceive soon after coming off the contraceptive pill may be deficient in some vitamins; this can affect the health of the developing baby. Another cause of nutritional deficiency is if the placenta is not fully functioning. This may occur if the baby is very late, as the placenta naturally starts to degenerate around the full term of pregnancy. Occasionally the placenta loses some of its capability before the end of pregnancy. This can cause a lack of oxygen and nutritional problems which slow down the baby's growth – or, if prolonged, even lead to severe pathologies.[27]

The imprint of experiences which relate to receiving nourishment in the womb are commonly held in the tissues around the umbilicus (belly button). It is primarily through the umbilicus that the baby experiences its life in the womb as either pleasant or toxic. If adequate nourishment is not received, the baby may be left with feelings such as getting its needs met is impossible, or that it isn't nurtured or loved. These feelings can become coupled with tissue contractions and lead to life statements such as 'Nobody loves me!' or 'I never get what I need!' or 'The world is a dirty place!'

Drugs

Many chemicals and drugs, such as antibiotics, pesticides, some hormones, alcohol and nicotine have been proven to be toxic to babies, and can adversely affect growth and development. Smoking has been linked to the birth of smaller babies and a higher incidence of infant mortality.[28] The chances of respiratory diseases such as asthma developing in childhood also increase if either parent smokes. It has also been found that alcohol abuse in pregnancy can cause malformation of the baby, and has been linked to learning difficulties later on. In cases where a mother is taking hard drugs such as cocaine or heroin, the baby is often born also suffering from this addiction.

Craniosacral work during pregnancy

Craniosacral therapy sessions can be of great benefit for a mother-to-be, helping to improve constitutional strength and addressing any stresses or traumas before their effects take root. It is also possible for the practitioner to palpate the baby's health while in the womb and to gently support its progress. Furthermore, treatment can help to relieve backache and relax the mother's pelvis. A well-balanced and relaxed pelvis can greatly ease the process of childbirth.

If the baby is in a breech position, the gentle encouragement of craniosacral work can help it to turn to a more easy presentation for birth. For example, Linda came for a session when she was at the full term of her pregnancy. However, her baby was in a breech position and she was feeling very concerned. When I put my hands on her abdomen, I noticed a stress pattern in her diaphragm and some contraction of the tissues in the right side of her pelvis. The baby also seemed to be affected by this inertia. After some gentle hands-on encouragement there was a much fuller sense of primary respiratory motion being expressed in the area. The next week I got a phone call from Linda. The same night of her treatment, her baby turned around into a position of normal presentation and she went straight into labour. She gave birth to a healthy 7-lb baby boy without any complications!

A *salutary example*

In the 1930s Margaret Meade, one of the pioneers of modern anthropology, came across a tribe who lived in the jungles of Papua and New Guinea. It seems that this tribe were especially aware of the significant effect of pregnancy and birth in shaping our lives. They were known as the 'peaceful people'; other, more aggressive tribes left them alone because they posed no threat. Margaret Meade found that when a woman of this tribe became pregnant, she was elevated to the position of a queen. The tribe would take care of all her needs so that she wouldn't suffer from any stress or strain. A mother-to-be was considered to be of great social importance because she was carrying the seed of the tribe in her womb. What was remarkable was that this tribe seemed to produce no traumatized babies, and were very harmonious in all their social interactions.

BIRTH

New technological advances have made birth less hazardous for mother and baby. However, the improvement in safety ceases at a certain point and thereafter the excessive use of machines and drugs creates problems and complications by interfering with the normal physiology of mother and baby.[29]
DR YEHUDI GORDON

A *baby's skull*

Being born is our first experience of meeting any strong physical resistance. On its journey into the world, a baby has to be literally squeezed through the narrow tunnel of its mother's pelvis. At this stage, an infant's skull is only partly formed and provides a superb balance of protection and pliability. This pliability is necessary to accommodate for the strong forces encountered in the birth canal.

The vault bones at the top of a baby's head largely consist of unfused membrane, which allows for enormous changes of shape. The places between the bones where this membrane remains soft are called the *fontanelles* (see Figure 10.1). The bones at the floor of the skull, the cranial base, consist largely of unfused cartilage. This cartilage also allows for a large degree of flexibility, and at the same time offers protection to the delicate organs at the base of the brain.[30]

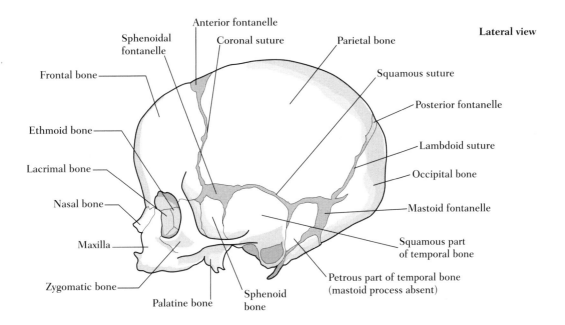

Figure 10.1: A baby's skull

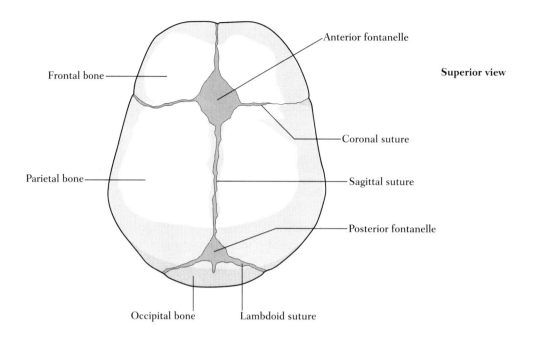

Figure 10.1 continued: A baby's skull

Many of the unfused bones of a baby's skull consist of separate parts. The fusion of these bones is a process which continues through childhood. Dr Viola Frymann noted that, 'Each portion of these bones may be regarded functionally as a separate bone, capable of moving in relation to its neighbor.'[31]

At birth, the frontal bone is in two parts, the temporal bones in three parts, the sphenoid bone in three parts, and the occiput in four parts (see Figure 10.2). The pelvis is also in three parts. As these bones meet with resistance during the birth process, they become liable to distortion. This frequently leads to the compression and irritation of underlying tissues. For example, if the different parts of the occiput become misshapen, the diameter of the foramen magnum may be reduced (see Figure 10.2). This can put pressure on the brainstem and the upper part of the spinal cord, both of which pass through this opening. Distortions can also cause irritation of the cranial nerves which emerge from smaller openings in or between the bones of the skull (see Effects on the nervous system, page 261).

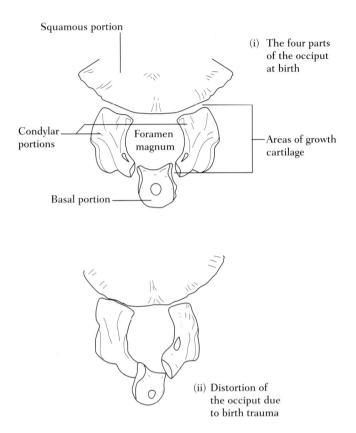

Squamous portion

(i) The four parts
of the occiput
at birth

Condylar portions

Foramen magnum

Areas of growth cartilage

Basal portion

(ii) Distortion of
the occiput due
to birth trauma

Figure 10.2: i) The four parts of the occiput at birth; ii) Distortion of the occiput

Cranial moulding

As a baby's head passes along the birth canal, it is squeezed into shapes which are determined by the contours of its mother's pelvis. These strong forces of compression can often last for several hours. The bones of its skull have to bend and overlap as they are squeezed together, in a process called *cranial moulding*. In addition, its body has to twist around, making a 90-degree rotation in order to gain exit. However, while this process is potentially traumatizing, it is also highly stimulating. These forces can be important in awakening the baby in preparation for its entry into the world.[32]

It seems that the manner of our birth is one of the greatest challenges we face. Most, but certainly not all babies are to some degree traumatized during this time. Nevertheless, many of these stresses are naturally rectified within the first 10 days, as the body's self-healing forces come into play. The underlying influence of primary respiratory motion, aided by the actions of suckling and crying, can sort out many of the less serious results of compression, allowing the baby's head to re-expand.

Unresolved inertia

However, stresses from birth commonly create inertial patterning that is at the root of various health problems. These structural strains cause difficulties which range from the more severe type, such as brain damage, epilepsy or autism, to less severe problems that are often considered to be 'normal'. Common symptoms include feeding difficulties, colic, excessive crying, irritability, poor sleep, developmental problems, emotional distress or ear or sinus problems.

Birth trauma can influence patterns of movement which are then permanently adopted. This is often first seen as asymmetries of motion or a strong preference in position. For example, if the baby only likes to feed on one side, it may suggest a neck strain. Or, parents may notice that their baby is uncomfortable when lying on one side. In many instances, these preferences are sufficient to cause an alteration in its pattern of growth.[33] According to Dr Ray Castellino, the patterns of motion adopted by a baby often reflect the events that occurred during a traumatic birth. He writes, 'This sequence of movements, postures and cranial patterns is later reproduced by the baby. The baby will move in ways and hold herself in positions reminiscent of her birth.'[34]

Emma's story

Emma was three years old when I first saw her. She suffered from repeated ear infections, 'glue ear' and partial deafness. Her sleep pattern was also very erratic and she would often wake suddenly, as if in a panic. Emma had been born after a long and difficult labour. She was stuck in the birth canal and in distress when the umbilical cord became caught around her neck. Eventually forceps were applied to the sides of her head to pull her out. Her mother had also been given an epidural injection to ease the pain.

Emma's head felt very hard, and her primary respiratory motion had a jerky quality, indicative of shock still held in her tissues. There was a lot of tightness and sensitivity in her cranial membranes and a compression of her left temporal bone (the organs of hearing are contained within the temporal bones). On the basis of these findings, I started treatment. Emma seemed to like the gentleness of craniosacral contact and even took my hands and placed them at the sides of her head, as if to say *'This* is where I need them!'

After the first two sessions, during which I worked with her cranial membranes and temporal bone, Emma's sleeping pattern showed some slight signs of improvement. Her mother also reported that Emma seemed less bothered by the discomfort in her ear. However, she then got another ear infection, which fortunately was not too serious. I advised her mother to try cutting down on dairy products in Emma's diet, which can help to prevent any excessive build-up of catarrh.

During the third treatment, Emma started to push her head against my hands, as if trying to resolve some of the tension in her skull. My hands provided her with some resistance to push against, and to Emma's great delight, she pushed right through and ended up in my arms. Emma slept for hours afterwards. When I saw her at the next visit, she looked brighter and more alert. Tests a couple of weeks later showed an 80 per cent improvement in her hearing. We followed up with another three treatments, which helped to further restore the expression of primary respiratory motion through her head. By the end of this course of treatment, Emma had made a complete recovery in all her symptoms.

Getting stuck

If a baby gets stuck in the birth canal, the degree of compression it experiences can be greatly intensified. If unresolved, this pattern of feeling stuck can repeat itself in later life. This commonly happens when such a person later finds themselves under stress or in an enclosed space. These situations can restimulate the memory (usually subconscious) of their birth panic. Life statements such as 'There's no way out!' or 'I can't get anywhere!' may consequently develop. Generally speaking, the earlier these inertial patterns can be addressed, the easier they are to treat.

Life and death patterns

Studies in Sweden have shown a very strong correlation between suicide and birth trauma. When conducting research in six Stockholm hospitals with patients who died from drug abuse, alcoholism or suicide, it was found that, more than any other risk factor, birth trauma was the greatest.[35] Furthermore, studies with adolescent suicide victims at the Karolensha Institute in Sweden showed that the type of trauma suffered at birth closely correlated with the method of suicide. For example, 2,900 cases in the survey who had died of asphyxiation had also suffered some kind of asphyxiation at birth. Out of those who had killed themselves by a mechanical procedure, many had also experienced a mechanical trauma at birth, such as being injured by forceps. The suicide victims who died from drug addiction had a strong correspondence with the administration of opiates and barbiturates at their birth.[36]

Brenda's story

Brenda, a successful businesswoman in her early thirties, suffered from claustrophobia. She had a great fear of flying, made all the worse by the fact that her work sometimes demanded that she travel. She would go into a panic, shaking uncontrollably, sweating profusely, heart-beat pounding, with rapid shallow breathing and tight neck muscles. Sometimes she would even vomit. She reported that she had had a long and difficult birth, during which time she'd become stuck in the birth canal and nearly died in the process.

Was her difficult birth the source of her distress? Perhaps this trauma was getting recapitulated whenever she felt trapped. On palpation, I found that there was a twist through the floor of her cranium and a compression pattern between her occiput and top vertebra of her neck. This may have been creating some irritation of her nervous system, perhaps including the vagus nerves (hence the rapid breathing and vomiting). We worked with these patterns with regular craniosacral therapy treatments over a period of about a year. Some sessions were very calm and soothing, whilst others involved strong involuntary movements of her body as the layers of shock held in her system were processed. Little by little, a re-organization of the tissues at the base of her skull took place and gradually Brenda no longer suffered from the same fearful reactions to enclosed spaces.

Asymmetries

Problems due to birth trauma can often be seen as asymmetries of the head and face. In fact, there are not many people who do not have marked differences between their right and left sides due to birth patterning. Any anomalies in your own skull can be seen by duplicating a photograph of your portrait onto two clear sheets of acetate, and then cutting each picture down the middle. This will give you two pictures of your left side and two pictures of your right side. If you then reverse one of the pictures of your left side and join it together with the other, you will have a photograph of yourself comprised of two left sides. Also join the two pictures of the right side of your head and face. You can then clearly see how different your face would look if made up of either two 'left' or two 'right' sides!

Natural childbirth

Within the last 20 years there has been a resurgence of interest in more natural approaches to childbirth. These approaches are intended to create an environment that is less traumatizing by making things as comfortable and pleasant as possible for both mother and baby. A natural childbirth also encourages both to trust their natural instincts. This is in contrast to practices still carried out in many hospitals where mothers are routinely made to stay on their backs to give birth, drugs are administered and the baby is often pulled out under force. The newborn then enters the glare of lights and the noisy excitement of the delivery room ... only for its umbilical cord to be cut straight away. It's hardly surprising that a newborn may contract to defend against these insensitivities.[37]

A more caring approach to delivering babies has been pioneered by obstetricians Dr Frederick Leboyer and Dr Michel Odent. Instead of becoming 'patients' who hand over all responsibility to the doctor, mothers are supported to take charge of the birthing process and to follow what *they* and *their baby* need. A mother is thus encouraged to choose her position, instead of taking it for granted that she has to lie on her back. In fact, it is usually much more difficult to give birth on one's back or semi-seated, as the sacrum and pelvis are less mobile in these positions. This can make it more difficult for the baby to emerge. A squatting position is generally easier for giving birth, because the sacrum and pelvis are free to open and the force of gravity is usefully employed.

It has also been found that giving birth in water, initially pioneered in Russia, can help to ease the pain of delivery and create a smooth transition for the baby as it leaves the watery environment of the womb to enter the world.[38]

Soft lighting, smooth and gentle sounds, warm air and loving and sensitive handling provide a fitting welcome for the newborn, and help to create an atmosphere of support.[39] If a mother is able to relax, the more likely it is that she will be able to stay in touch with her natural instincts and have an easier birth without the use of medical intervention. The role of the father is also of great importance to provide support and safekeeping. A father's presence and engagement with the birth of his child can profoundly contribute to the sanctuary of the environment. When handled with sensitivity, an experience of excitement, joy and bliss can play as much a part in the process of childbirth as any of the challenges that mother and baby face.[40]

CAUSES OF COMPLICATIONS

*Learn to respect this sacred moment of birth, as fragile, as fleeting, as
elusive as dawn. The child is there, hesitant, tentative, unsure which way
he's about to go. He stands between two worlds.*[41]
FREDERICK LEBOYER

Whether or not a baby has a traumatic entry into the world (and remains traumatized) is
determined by a number of factors. We'll now take a look at each of these factors in turn.

The shape and size of the mother's pelvis

Some pelvic shapes are much easier to be born through, while others provide more of a chal-
lenge. If the mother's pelvis is very narrow or more triangular in shape, the baby may be
unable to easily navigate a way through. The size of the pelvis is also of critical importance.
With some pelvic types, a caesarean section is often carried out prior to the onset of labour to
prevent complications (see below).

The size of the baby

Babies vary greatly in size and, of course, the larger the baby the more difficulty it can have
moving through the confines of the birth canal. Naturally, if the mother's pelvis is also large
this is of less significance. The average baby weighs about 7 lb (3.175 kg); any baby who is
over about 9 lb (4.082 kg) is generally considered large. A large baby is more likely to get
stuck and may also have difficulty getting its shoulders out once the head has been born.

The position of the baby

The position of the baby as it passes through the birth canal also determines the ease of delivery. Certain positions make for an easier exit, while others can create difficulties. The easiest
position in which to be born is head-first; this is the most common presentation. Less strain is
also caused when the baby moves through the birth canal in what is called a 'posterior presentation'. This is when the baby's face moves down past the mother's sacrum as it gains exit
(see Figure 10.3). An 'anterior presentation' is when the back of the baby's head moves past
the mother's sacrum. It is more common for a baby to get stuck when in this position. The
angle at which the baby's head meets the pelvis at the onset of labour is also important. Its

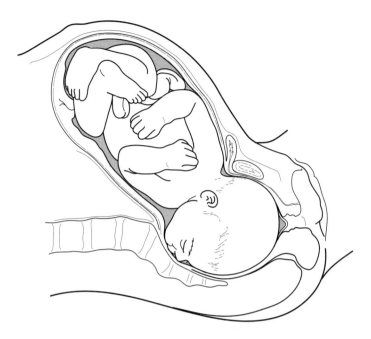

Figure 10.3: Posterior presentation – the baby's face moves past the mother's sacrum

head is ideally tucked in against its chest, which provides the smallest possible diameter for it to pass into the birth canal. It also helps if the baby's head is at a slight angle, rather than full-on, as it starts its descent.

Perhaps the most difficult way to be born is from a breech position, where the baby comes out bottom-first. In this instance, the forces of compression tend to enter the baby's body from the bottom up, and its hips and pelvis often suffer from strain. Furthermore, the baby's head doesn't undergo the benefits of proper moulding. Other positions of birth, such as shoulder-first, are less common, but can also create patterns of strain or injury.

Length of labour

A labour that is very long (over 15 hours) subjects the baby to sustained forces of compression, which often increase in pressure if the baby is stuck. This is more likely to overwhelm the baby, and raises the chances of traumatization. The force of the mother's contractions together with the resistance provided by her pelvis can create localized areas of compression and distortion in the pliable tissues of the baby. These patterns can remain, and are frequently seen in the adult who comes for craniosacral treatment.

In a very quick labour (under six hours), the forces of the mother's pelvic contractions are often very strong and fast. As a result, the baby's head may not have time to mould gently and slowly, which can lead to an experience of shock held in the tissues. Furthermore, it is likely that the baby will feel considerable fear. This may cause irritability, difficulty in settling and a wide range of other symptoms.

Umbilical difficulties

In some cases the umbilical cord becomes twisted around the baby's body during delivery, which may delay its progress through the birth canal. If the cord becomes compressed (or if the placenta separates early), it can cut off the baby's oxygen supply. Even a brief interruption of the supply of oxygen may leave the baby in a state of distress or shock. A steady oxygen supply is required for the survival of the brain, and any stoppage of more than a few minutes can lead to damage and the onset of cerebral palsy. This is usually marked by a severe loss of motility in the baby's cranial bones and central nervous system.

The umbilical cord can sometimes get caught around the baby's neck, causing strangulation and making it hard for the baby to emerge fully. Neck problems and sensitivity in the area of the throat are often the result.

When I was treating the region around the umbilicus of a 29-year-old patient, he started to feel that he was being strangled. When he explored this sensation a little further, he felt the urge to struggle, but then found that the more he struggled the worse his feeling of being strangled became. Although there is no evidence to connect these events, his experience fitted in with the way his umbilical cord became caught around his neck when he was born.

Umbilical shock

In general birthing practice, the umbilical cord is cut straight after the baby is born. However, ideally it should remain intact until it has stopped pulsating, which is often five minutes or more after birth. Only when it stops pulsating is it no longer in use. The baby can then, without shock or danger, settle down to breathing on its own.[42] If the cord is cut too soon it may cause the baby trauma, which is often retained in the tissues around its umbilicus.

My own experience of umbilical shock is an illustration. During a craniosacral treatment my therapist started to sense a place of inertia in the region of my belly button. When she made contact with this area, I experienced a strong sensation, as if I had been hit in the abdomen – a feeling that made me want to groan. This sensation stayed with me while my therapist followed the pattern in my tissues to a state of balanced tension. After some pulsations and twitches in my abdomen, everything seemed to settle and I started to feel quite drowsy. At this point my therapist cradled my head while I rested and fell asleep. I found this to be extraordinarily comforting, as this is just what didn't happen when I was born. I awoke feeling deeply healed and very calm.

Caesarean section

A surgical birth is called a *caesarean section*, after Julius Caesar, who was born in this way. A caesarean section is often advised by doctors if there is some difficulty with having a vaginal birth. While a baby born by caesarean section doesn't have to undergo all the compressive forces of conventional childbirth, this procedure nevertheless does carry problems of its own. The type of problems depend on whether it is an 'elected' or an emergency caesarean section. An elected caesarean is one that is carried out before the mother goes into labour. It may be performed if the mother has an illness which makes a vaginal birth difficult, or if her pelvis is too small or narrow to accommodate the passage of her baby. An emergency caesarean is carried out if a difficulty arises which puts either mother or baby in danger once labour has started.

A baby who is born by an elected caesarean is deprived of the positive benefits provided by the process of moulding as it passes through the birth canal. These babies are often less responsive as a result. They can end up clingy and often need constant engagement or something to push against in later life. A caesarean section also produces a sudden change in pressure from the environment of the womb to the outside world. This may result in the baby experiencing shock and create a contractile response in its tissues. Consequently, the heads of caesarean babies often feel very hard and are more immobile.

With an emergency caesarean, the baby may be traumatized from the effects of the complication that created the need for surgical intervention. This is in addition to the effects of the pressure change described above. Furthermore, it may not be easy to disengage the baby if it is deeply wedged in the mother's pelvis, and the doctor often has to pull hard to get it out. Nevertheless, the intervention of a caesarean section can save lives.

Age of the baby at birth

A baby born at the full-term of pregnancy generally has a better chance of an easier birth. At this point its skull has developed to an optimal point of flexibility for a smooth birth and is also strong enough to provide protection to the brain. However, the skull of a baby who is over 40 weeks may be further developed and therefore harder. Consequently, it may be less accommodating for the forces of childbirth.

With the advancement of medical science, babies can now survive from a very early stage of prematurity. In recent years it is not unusual for babies as young as 27 weeks to pull through, even though they may require considerable medical intervention. Babies younger than 32 weeks need a ventilator to supply them with oxygen, and food has to be provided intravenously. Even the lungs of babies who are only a few weeks premature may be placed under strain in the outside world because they have not fully developed. This is sometimes palpated as a loss of primary respiratory motion in the chest. The bones of premature babies are still very soft and therefore give less protection during childbirth. Furthermore, the effects of gravity after birth can cause their skulls to flatten when they sleep, a phenomenon often seen in the skulls of premature babies.

Interventions used

A natural childbirth, in the familiar surroundings of home and without any intervention, is definitely the ideal. Babies who have this kind of birth tend to be more alert, more co-ordinated and happier. Nevertheless, if there are complications during childbirth, a quick response using medical intervention can be a vital life-saver. However, in modern hospitals interventions are frequently used defensively, in the fear that something may happen, even if it hasn't actually happened. This mentality seems to stem from a deep-seated mistrust of our natural instincts and capabilities, and from a lack of recognition that childbirth is fundamentally a natural process. It seems that the doctor's concern about litigation if something does go wrong is increasingly the motivation for the use of invasive treatment.

Drugs administered to the mother, either during pregnancy or childbirth, may also enter the baby's bloodstream and have a deep effect. Furthermore, they may stay within the baby's system for many years after birth. Pethidine (Demorol in the US) is one such painkilling drug frequently prescribed during labour. Babies born with this drug tend to be sleepy and irritable, and their tissues often feel sluggish on palpation.

Epidurals are relatively less harmful to the baby, but the mother's pelvis is numbed as a result, so she may then need the help of further interventions, such as forceps, to help the baby come out. Epidurals also often create longer-term back pain in the mother.

The use of gas and air for pain relief seems to create less severe reactions, but still often leads to a fragmentation of function in the baby and a tendency to dissociate.

There is much evidence to suggest that the onset of labour is actually initiated by the baby who, when it is ready, triggers the release of the hormone oxytocin in the mother.[43] Oxytocin causes the uterus to contract. However, sometimes drugs are prescribed to produce contractions artificially if the baby is overdue. As a result, these babies are literally pushed out at a pace which is too fast for them.

If a baby gets stuck during the later stages of labour, forceps or a *ventouse suction* appliance may be used to bring it out. Forceps are generally applied to the sides of the baby's head, sometimes with a lot of pressure, which pulls on the tissues and causes bruising. However, if used skilfully forceps can save distress and do not necessarily cause a problem.

A ventouse appliance employs a cup which is attached on top of the baby's head and used to suck it out of the pelvis. This often creates significant stress and a distortion of the baby's head.

Replaying complications

Keith was a 25-year-old man who came for craniosacral sessions, suffering from depression and recurrent back pain. He often struggled, with great effort, to achieve things in his life, but then would give up, feeling that he couldn't succeed. This may have been a replay of his birth trauma. His mother was given drugs to induce the onset of labour when Keith was about a week overdue. As a result he was pushed out, drugged with painkillers and finally pulled with forceps, so that he was born hardly under his own steam. Later in life Keith would repeatedly set himself tasks but be overcome by feelings of weakness and a lack of confidence, so that he was unable to complete them. Sadly, Keith discontinued treatment before he was able to find the resources to move through this pattern.

Parents' health

The health of both parents at the time of conception is considered to have an important influence on the developing baby's constitutional strength. The health of the mother is particularly critical during pregnancy and childbirth. Most acute illnesses are generally not a problem for the baby, but if the mother suffers from a serious condition or infection, it may affect the baby's progress.[44] For example, the consequences of contracting German measles (rubella) during pregnancy are well known and may cause deafness in the baby. Morning sickness is a frequent symptom during the earlier stages of pregnancy, but this will normally not have any adverse influence on the baby. However, persistent vomiting which continues throughout pregnancy may affect the baby's available supply of nutrition and result in a slowing of its growth.

Order of birth

Once the birth canal has been stretched by a first child, it will usually be easier for it to stretch again with any subsequent birth. Therefore, later children will often benefit from the pathway 'pioneered' by their older brothers or sisters. Complications more frequently affect a first child because the mother's pelvis is less flexible, and perhaps also because she may be more anxious the first time. However, if there is any scar tissue from a previous birth it may provide resistance to the passage of a later baby.

Bonding

The process of bonding between a baby and its parents starts right at the beginning of pregnancy. The feeling of nurturing that a baby finds from its parents is important for the activity of its self-healing capabilities. Once a baby is born, many of the less severe results of traumatization are naturally resolved. At this point, the love and support that a baby receives can greatly enhance its ability to heal. However, if this bonding doesn't take place, the baby may be less able to thrive.

Breastfeeding is usually an important part of the bonding process and is one of the key ways that a baby will feel nurtured. Interestingly, studies have shown that if babies are left undisturbed on their mother's abdomen directly after birth, they will naturally start to make their own way to the nipple and latch on for their first feed.[45,46] They innately know what to do. Trusting these natural instincts permits the baby to discover that it is possible to go for what it needs, and to get its needs met. However, it has also been demonstrated that even a brief separation of the newborn from its mother after birth has a strong effect on the success of the first feed. The use of drugs and other medical interventions is another factor that has been shown to inhibit the baby's ability to suckle.[47]

WORKING WITH BABIES AND CHILDREN

*It is the more obscure, the so-called minimal injuries of no apparent
clinical significance that too often go undetected and that are so often
responsible for problems of development and growth during periods of
infancy, childhood and adolescence.*[48]
DR A. G. CATHIE

There is a strong case for every baby to be checked by a craniosacral therapist soon after birth. Details of the pregnancy and birth may give valuable clues about the origin of any difficulties, and so may be of particular interest to the practitioner. As many of the problems that result from a difficult birth or earlier trauma are treatable, much suffering in later life can be prevented. The range of possible symptoms is quite extensive, but some of the most typical problems are outlined below.

Traumatization

Initially, the craniosacral therapist checks for any sign of traumatization. This may show up as a difficulty in maintaining eye contact, or signs of withdrawal, dissociation, stress, excessive crying or irritability. In extreme cases the baby may have entered a *hypotonic* state. This is marked by flaccidity of the tissues and lack of potency in the rhythms of primary respiratory motion. It occurs in circumstances where the baby's physiology has suffered a large degree of overwhelm and traumatization. As a result, the baby may have literally given up. This state often underlies tendencies towards emotional depression, a lack of confidence and resignation in later life. In many of these cases, any kind of contact is experienced as painful because it reminds the baby of the distress still residing deep within its system. This kind of situation can also be at the root of autism.

Building up potency resources is the first step in the treatment of these babies.

Effects on the nervous system

At birth, the human brain is only about one-quarter of its adult weight.[49] Thus, the majority of brain growth occurs once we are out of the womb. The bones of the skull and the reciprocal tension membranes help to determine the shape of the brain as it grows. If inertial patterns are retained in these tissues, it can affect the way this growth occurs. As a result, the primary respiratory motion of the nervous system may be disturbed, causing irritation of the brain and cranial nerves. Functioning of the nervous system may also be upset if it remains in a state of shock after a long or difficult birth.

Pressure on the cranial nerves often results from compression of the small openings through which they gain exit from the skull. For example, if the suture between the occiput and temporal bones is compressed, the vagus nerve may become irritated – colic is commonly the result.

It's often fairly simple to aid the decompression of this region and remove the cause of irritation. This is one of the occasions when an immediate relief of symptoms can occur with craniosacral treatment.

Heartbeat irregularities, respiratory or other digestive upsets also commonly result if the vagus nerve is compressed. Furthermore, the same opening in the suture, the jugular foramen, contains the glossopharyngeal nerve which supplies some of the muscles of the throat and the largest salivary gland. If it becomes irritated, difficulties with swallowing and feeding can result.

Similarly, problems with suckling may occur if the nearby hypoglossal nerve becomes irritated, commonly due to inertial patterns which affect the occiput. If the baby's suckling is weak, more air tends to be drawn in, which can further contribute to wind and colicky pains.

Pressure on other cranial nerves may cause eye problems such as involuntary movements or a squint. Ear infections, hearing difficulties and 'glue ear' can all result from inertia involving the temporal bone and resultant cranial nerve irritation. The eustachian tube (which regulates pressure in the ear) may become blocked, leading to a build-up of pressure and a tendency to ear infections. All of these are detectable by palpation and can be amenable to treatment.

Cranial compression

Any excessive cranial moulding retained from childbirth may pressurize or even damage underlying nerve tissue. Cerebral palsy may have a number of causes but, according to Dr John Upledger, included in these are 'abnormal tensions of the dura mater membrane and/or jamming of some of the sutures of the skull vault'.[50] This jamming frequently involves the coronal suture located at the top of the head between the frontal bone and the parietal bones, and is often the consequence of a traumatic birth. Some of these cases can show improvement with the use of craniosacral treatment.[51] Dr Upledger also describes a 'severe membranous (dural) restriction of the craniosacral system' commonly found in autistic children.[52]

Sleep disturbances, headaches or even head-banging may be due to an increase of pressure in the baby's head. Thumb-sucking is often an unconscious attempt to try to free restrictions which involve the hard palate. Inertia held in the jaw and hard palate will often be the cause of an overcrowding of teeth and the development of dental problems. Sinus problems can result from compressions which involve the bones at the front of the head. The *sphenopalatine ganglion* is a nerve bundle located between the sphenoid bone and the hard palate. A runny nose, problems with the tear ducts, hay fever or facial pain may result if this ganglion is irritated.

Problems with co-ordination

Other signs of traumatization include jerky and uncoordinated movements, or if the baby doesn't like to have its legs raised, for example when its nappy (diaper) is changed. Sometimes babies develop a lack of orientation which is shown if they are unable to focus their attention towards one side.

Trauma may also be indicated if the baby's normal milestones of development are not being met. For example, the baby may be late in its ability to sit, crawl, walk or talk. Or, later on, other symptoms such as learning difficulties, dyslexia or hyperactivity may develop.

Body patterns

Spinal curvatures may result from compressions which occurred as the baby twisted through the birth canal to gain exit. Inertia affecting the chest and ribs can restrict the drainage of lymphatic fluid and the functioning of the thymus gland, important parts of the immune system. This can predispose the baby to recurrent infections. Asthmatic babies and children often show signs of birth trauma which involved compression of the chest or a loss of oxygen during childbirth. The nerve centres controlling the lungs are located towards the back of the brain and can also be affected by compression. Tension held in the abdomen and diaphragm is another cause of colic in babies. Craniosacral treatment often helps to restore order and balance by facilitating primary respiratory motion in these areas. This can improve the circulation of lymphatic fluids through the chest, encourage more flexibility in the muscles, bones and internal organs, and remove the causes of nerve irritation.

Toxicity

The effects of parents' smoking or the use of drugs are often palpable in the baby's rhythms of primary respiratory motion. These babies will often have a sluggishness of movement, a lack of fluid drive and, typically, their tissues will have an 'uneasy' feel. However, the restoration of a full and balanced expression of the Breath of Life can be encouraged, helping the circulatory systems to dispose of any toxins. According to the old Chinese saying, 'Running water clears itself.'

James' story

James was a year old when his mother brought him for craniosacral treatment. He was still not sitting up, his movements were wobbly and he had recently been diagnosed by his paediatrician with 'floppy muscle tone'. His right eyelid drooped and his head was lumpy and uneven. He was also very irritable, with long periods of crying and frequent tantrums. The first sign I had of his arrival was a loud and constant screaming coming from the waiting room!

James had been born five days overdue, after being induced. In addition, his mother had been given Pethidine to ease the pain. Although there were no major problems during the pregnancy, his mother had experienced a lot of anxiety because of her own mother's illness. While examining him, James entered a screaming tantrum which continued until he went blue in the face despite all efforts to comfort him. Although I was hardly able to make physical contact before he became disturbed, it was clear that his whole head felt very tight, his nervous system was in a state of shock and that the bones and membranes at the base of his skull had become distorted.

During his second visit, I again negotiated contact with James and was able to sense a little more. I noticed a particular strain pattern involving the frontal bone, which was locked in a position of torsion. I again had to stop treatment when he started another episode of screaming. As James found it so difficult to tolerate contact, I knew that we would have to work slowly and sensitively.

We met again the following week and this time I was able to make contact for a little longer and encourage a little more space at his frontal bone. Subsequently, his mother remarked that there was an improvement in his temperament and his drooping eyelid was less pronounced on some days. Meanwhile, a report from the neurologist stated that no abnormalities could be detected for James' condition and gave him the all-clear. This allowed us free reign to explore the craniosacral causes of his distress.

The following treatment was again largely spent at James' frontal bone, and some more decompression of this area was encouraged. His mother then reported that he was starting to sit up and was putting on weight. During the next treatment I started to work at James' sphenoid bone and the orbit of his right eye. However, within a few minutes he again started screaming until he was blue in the face, so I decided just to play with him for a while until he settled. Nevertheless, after this the drooping of his eyelid further improved.

Two weeks later I worked with a strong pattern of inertia which showed itself in James' membrane system. His falx cerebri (vertical partition of the head) had become twisted and this was interfering with the ability of the bones at the base of his skull to express their motion. During treatment James gave a little shudder and these tissues started to open up. Following this, he seemed a lot happier. Not only were his legs straightening, but he was also starting to take his weight on them. One month later James was taking his first steps and beginning to play with other children.

Treatment of babies and children

The primary respiratory system of a baby or child can be very finely balanced and delicate. Therefore, treatment needs to be applied with plenty of care and negotiation. Babies and children tend to respond quickly to craniosacral treatment, perhaps because they have accumulated fewer layers of conditioning which can get in the way. However, they may also have difficulty in keeping still for any length of time, and so treatments tend to be applied in small doses. Trust with a therapist often needs to be developed, and so it is quite useful to have a few toys to hand which can be used to befriend the child. Sometimes it is necessary to follow a young child around the room while playing and giving a treatment at the same time! Infants can often more easily be treated while they are nursing.

Only direct methods of treatment are generally used when working with the cranial bones of babies or young children (see Chapter 7, Direct approaches, page 168). This is because their sutures have not yet properly formed. As sutures help to determine the allowable motion of a cranial bone, if a practitioner facilitates its motion the boundary to how far it can move is often unclear. Therefore, with an indirect approach (i.e. following a strain pattern into its preferred direction) tissues may just keep moving into their trauma pattern. This may cause retraumatization of the baby. Therefore, working with the potency in the fluids and encouraging space and disengagement of compressed tissues are the most effective treatment approaches for babies and young children. In this way, distortions within cranial bones can be gently remoulded and their contours gradually normalized.[53]

Treatment for mothers

Mothers too can benefit from craniosacral work to support rebalancing after childbirth. Treatment can help strains in the pelvis or sacrum return to a normal position and ease any residual low backache. Furthermore, pulls or strains which affect the mother's nervous system can contribute to feelings of tiredness and post-natal depression.

Sometimes the uterus becomes malpositioned from giving birth; a situation that may cause dragging pains in the pelvis. These patterns are often helped by craniosacral treatment.

Transforming repetitive cycles

Working with mothers, babies and children is perhaps one of the most rewarding aspects of craniosacral practice. It's a particular joy to see the progress of infants as they find increased levels of integration and aliveness. As a culture it seems that we often become trapped in repetitive cycles of conditioning and suffering which have their origins in the unresolved traumatic experiences of birth. This is perhaps the same process that our parents, and their parents before them underwent, too. As Dr Leboyer perceives,

> *... How naive, how innocent to imagine no trace will remain;*
> *that one could emerge unscathed from such an experience.*
> *The scars are everywhere: in our flesh, our bones, our backs,*
> *our nightmares, our madness, and all the insanity, the folly*
> *of this world – its tortures, its wars, its prisons.*[54]

While we may have made huge progressions technologically and materially, a fragmentation in the way we function and consequent ill-health is still very much a part of our lives. However, a great deal of suffering may be prevented by transforming cycles of trauma and inertia at an early point in life. What then would be the kind of world in which we live?

GLOSSARY

Active alert	a state of heightened awareness triggered when there is a possibility of danger
Allopathic	a system of medicine where remedies or drugs are prescribed to produce a condition that is the opposite of those produced by the disease being treated
Alzheimer's disease	a degenerative condition of the central nervous system which causes dementia
Anatomy	the study of the structure of the body
Anterior	towards the front of the body
Aqueduct of Silvius	a long thin channel which connects the third and fourth ventricles of the brain
Arachnoid	the middle layer of the meningeal membrane system which surrounds the central nervous system. It resembles a spider's web.
Arachnoid villi	microscopic finger-like projections of tissue in the arachnoid layer of the meningeal membrane system. Cerebrospinal fluid is reabsorbed through the arachnoid villi into venous sinuses.
Asthma	a respiratory condition which causes wheezing and shortness of breath, marked by contraction of the bronchial tubes. Sufferers usually have more difficulty in breathing out than breathing in.
Autism	a condition (which usually begins at birth) marked by disorders of communication, withdrawal from contact and self-absorption
Autonomic nervous system	the part of the nervous system which controls the functioning of the body's organs and which is not typically under voluntary control. It is comprised of the sympathetic and parasympathetic branches.
Axis (plural: axes)	an imaginary line around which a structure moves. *Horizontal* or *transverse axis* – an axis which goes from side to side. *Anterior-posterior axis* – an axis which goes from front to back. *Vertical axis* – an axis which goes from top to bottom.
Ayurveda (adj. Ayurvedic)	the traditional medical system practised in the Indian sub-continent
Basal ganglia	groups of nerve cell bodies in the cerebral hemispheres and upper brainstem involved with motor co-ordination
Bevel	the type of joint or suture which has an angled surface and that mainly allows for a gliding motion
Biodynamic potency/ force	the basic energy of wellness, the intrinsic force produced by the Breath of Life which is conveyed in the fluids of the body
Biokinetic potency/ force	the added forces of stress and conditioning, which the biodynamic forces have to accommodate for

Biosphere	the whole sphere of physiological activity of a person, including physical and energetic processes and their interaction with the environment
Boundary	i) the demarcation between patient and practitioner, ii) the physiological edge of a tissue's pattern of motion, before any strain is added to make it move further
Breath of Life	a term used by Dr W. G. Sutherland to describe our essential life-force; an invisible element, a 'fluid within a fluid' which contains an innate intelligence. It is essentially expressed as a slow tide-like rhythm, the long tide, which then unfolds into the faster rhythms of the mid-tide and the cranial rhythmic impulse.
Caduceus	the entwining energies which are located along the central 'rod' of the spine, used as a symbol of the medical profession
Caesarean section	delivery of a baby from its mother's pelvis by abdominal surgery
Cartilage	a type of fibrous connective tissue, out of which much of the bony skeleton becomes formed. This resilient tissue lines many of the freely movable joints of the body.
Cerebellum	part of the brain, located at the lower, posterior part of the skull. It consists of a central area and two lateral hemispheres, and is chiefly concerned with balance, movement and muscle tone.
Cerebral palsy	a group of disorders caused by damage to areas of the brain which produce or affect movement (i.e. motor functions).
Cerebrospinal fluid (C.S.F.)	a transparent, slightly yellowish fluid which bathes the central nervous system. Acts as a conveyor of potency, and called by Dr A. T. Still 'the highest known element in the body'.
Cerebrum	the main portion of the brain, consisting of the cortex – which is formed of two lateral hemispheres, connected in the middle. Responsible for conscious thought and behaviour.
Chakra	a Sanskrit word referring to a centre or gateway through which energy or vital force is distributed. It literally translates as 'wheel'.
Choroid plexus (plural: plexi)	projections in the blood capillary system of the brain which produce cerebrospinal fluid and secrete it into the ventricles
Clinoid processes	small projections of bone on the upper surface of the sphenoid bone which provide the anterior attachments for the tentorium cerebelli and which surround the sella turcica (saddle), housing the pituitary gland
Coccyx	the small tail bones at the base of the spine, formed of two to four bones, which are usually fused
Collagen fibres	microscopic hollow fibres made of protein, contained within connective tissues and which allow for the passage of small amounts of cerebrospinal fluid

Colic	acute abdominal pain. Can sometimes be caused by irritation of the vagus nerve.
Compression	the movement or forcing of structures closer towards each other
Connective tissue	tissues which surround and connect different parts of the body. Fascia is one important type of connective tissue.
Core link	a term coined by Dr W. G. Sutherland referring to the spinal dural membrane which connects the sacrum to the cranium
Cortex	literally means 'outer layer'. Often used to refer to the hemispheres of the brain (cerebral cortex).
Cortisol	a hormone secreted by the adrenal glands as part of the body's response to stress. Helps to provide energy and is an anti-inflammatory.
Coupling	the association of an emotion or attitude with a physiological response in the body
Cranial base	the floor of the skull which is embryologically formed from cartilage. Often used to refer to the sphenoid and occiput.
Cranial concept	the philosophy and practice developed by Dr W. G. Sutherland which involves an appreciation of the rhythmic motions produced by the Breath of Life, and the significance of the primary respiratory system for the maintenance of balance and health
Cranial osteopathy	the study and practice of the cranial concept which is considered to be a part of osteopathic health care practised by osteopaths
Cranial rhythmic impulse (C.R.I.)	the outermost expression of the Breath of Life, which has a rhythmic motion of an average 6–12 cycles per minute. Sometimes shortened to 'cranial rhythm'. Can be palpated throughout the body.
Craniosacral concept	same as 'cranial concept'
Craniosacral motion	the different motions produced in the fluids and tissues of the body as a result of the cranial rhythmic impulse
Craniosacral rhythm	same as the 'cranial rhythmic impulse'
Craniosacral system	same as 'primary respiratory mechanism'
Craniosacral therapy	a system of holistic health care which places an emphasis on supporting the expressions of primary respiratory motion. This term was coined by Dr John Upledger.
Cranium	the bones of the skull
Crista galli	a small projection at the top of the ethmoid bone, providing the attachment for the anterior aspect of the falx cerebri. Resembles a cock's comb.
Decompression	the movement of structures away from each other; the creation of space between structures
Direct approach	a treatment approach which facilitates motion away from the direction of preference of an inertial pattern

Direction of preference	the direction in which tissues move most easily, as the result of an inertial pattern
Disengagement	the separation of two bones which have become compressed together
Dissociation	a fragmentation of function which happens in states of overwhelm as part of a protective response; a state of being 'out of touch'
DNA (deoxyribonucleic acid)	coiled protein strands within the nucleus of a cell containing the information of our inherited (genetic) tendencies
Dura mater	the tough and relatively inelastic outer layer of the membranous lining which surrounds the central nervous system. It is composed of two layers of tissue, largely fused together.
Dyslexia	a condition marked by difficulty with comprehending written language
Elastin fibres	one of the constituents of connective tissue, made of fibres of protein. They are found in different connective tissues in varying quantities, providing varying degrees of flexibility and elasticity.
Embryo	the developing human being from about age two weeks to eight weeks after conception, during which time all the major body structures are formed
Embryological	pertaining to the period of embryonic development
Embryonic disc	a flattened area in the fertilized egg in which the first traces of the embryo are seen
Endocrine	pertaining to the glands and secretions of the hormonal system
Endorphin	a painkilling chemical secreted by the brain
Energy cyst	a walled-off area of kinetic energy which develops in response to a physical trauma whose force the body has been unable to dissipate
Entrapped force vector	same as 'energy cyst'
Epilepsy	a collection of transient symptoms characterized by seizures, caused by abnormal electrical activity of the brain
Ethmoid bone	a light, airy bone of the cranium, located behind the brow and forming part of the walls of the nasal cavity and the orbit
Eustachian tube	the canal which links the middle ear and the back part of the mouth just above the soft palate. Regulates pressure in the ear.
Exaggeration	the encouragement of tissues further into their inertial pattern
Exhalation	the phase of primary respiratory motion during which there is a receding motion towards the lower part of the body and a narrowing from side to side. Within the cranial rhythmic impulse, it coincides with the extension/internal rotation phase.
Extension	a movement that increases the angle between two structures. Used to describe the motion of single midline bones in the exhalation phase of the cranial rhythmic impulse.

External rotation	a rotation away from the midline. Used to describe the motion of paired structures in the inhalation phase of the cranial rhythmic impulse.
Facilitated segment	a hypersensitive segment of the spinal cord, which fires nerve impulses with a minimum of stimulation
Falx cerebelli	the smaller vertical partition formed of dura in the reciprocal tension membrane system, dividing the two hemispheres of the cerebellum
Falx cerebri	the larger vertical partition in the reciprocal tension membrane system, formed of dura and shaped like a sickle, which divides the two hemispheres of the cerebrum
Fascia	a type of connective tissue which covers, supports and connects all the different structures of the body, forming a continuous network throughout the body
Fight or flight response	a physiological response to threat or danger during which the body is put on alert and its resources are mobilized to either fight or run away
Flexion	a movement which decreases the angle between two structures. Used to describe the motion of single midline bones in the inhalation phase of the cranial rhythmic impulse.
Fluid drive	the strength or force behind the longitudinal fluctuation of cerebrospinal fluid, due to the amount of potency it carries
Foetus	the developing baby from the end of the embryonic period of pregnancy to the time of birth
Fontanelle	a membrane in the vault portion of the skull of a foetus or young child, covering areas which have not yet hardened into bone
Foramen magnum	the large opening at the base of the skull, located in the occipital bone, providing a passage for the lower part of the brainstem and upper part of the spinal cord
Force vector	the pathway in which kinetic energy enters the body as a result of a physical trauma
Frontal bone	the bone that forms the forehead and the upper part of the orbits
Fulcrum	a point around which motion takes place. *Inertial fulcrum* – a place of stasis where the Breath of Life is unable to find expression and containing unresolved forces which organize patterns of restriction in the body. *Practitioner fulcrum* – a focus around which the practitioner can operate and orientate.
Ganglion (plural: ganglia)	a collection or bundle of nerve cell bodies. (Also, a form of benign tumour located in a muscle tendon.)
Gastritis	inflammation of the stomach
Glossopharyngeal nerve	a cranial nerve which exits the skull through the jugular foramen. It supplies some of the muscles of the throat, the taste buds and the largest salivary gland.

Glue ear	a build-up of fluid and catarrh in the ear which more frequently affects young children, due to obstruction of the eustachian (auditory) tube
Groundswell	the centrifugal and centripedal motion which is produced as the Breath of Life emerges from the ground of dynamic stillness
Healing crisis	an acute reaction occurring as part of a healing process, when the body attempts to dissipate the elements which cause and maintain disease
Hologram	a three-dimensional image produced when lasers are shone through a photographic plate. The whole image is encoded within each part of the plate.
Homeostasis	the state of inner physiological balance which is maintained by numerous mechanisms of the body
Homunculus	an effigy, often used to illustrate the proportional amounts of the brain employed to receive information from specific regions of the body (sensory) or to control the functioning (motor) of specific regions of the body
Hormone	a chemical secretion which has a specific regulatory effect in the body, mostly produced by the glands of the hormonal (endocrine) system
Hyperactivity	excessive activity which is marked by fidgetiness, excitability, impulsiveness, irritability and a short attention span
Hypoglossal nerve	cranial nerve which exits from the skull through a small opening in the occipital bone, supplying the muscles of the tongue and involved with a baby's ability to suckle
Hypothalamus	a small, yet vitally important region of the brain which regulates and integrates many functions of the body, including the autonomic nervous system and the hormonal system. Sometimes referred to as 'the brain of the brain'.
Hypotonic	loss of tone in tissues
Immune system	the collection of organs involved with the body's ability to fight infection
Ilium (plural: ilia; adj. iliac)	the bone which forms the upper portion and side of the pelvis
Indirect approach	a treatment approach in which inertial patterns are followed into their direction of preference
Inferior	towards the lower part of the body
Inhalation	the phase of primary respiratory motion during which there is a rising tide towards the upper part of the body and a widening from side to side. Within the cranial rhythmic impulse, it coincides with the flexion/external rotation phase.
Inherent treatment plan	the treatment priorities of the patient's own physiology
Internal jugular veins	a pair of veins through which 95 per cent of fluid drains from the cranium, passing through the jugular foramen

Internal rotation	a rotation towards the midline. Used to describe the motion of paired structures in the exhalation phase of the cranial rhythmic impulse.
Interstitial	between tissues or in the spaces within tissues
Intraosseous	within a bone
Involuntary mechanism	same as 'primary respiratory mechanism'
Jugular foramen (plural: foramina)	a small hole located (both sides) at the base of the skull in the suture between the temporal and occipital bones, through which the internal jugular vein, vagus nerve, glossopharyngeal nerve and spinal accessory nerve all pass
Kinetic	relating to the property of motion or force
Lacrimal bones	small paired bones located at the inner borders of the orbit. Contain the tear ducts.
Lamina terminalis	a sheet of tissue which forms the anterior wall of the third ventricle. Acts as the natural fulcrum for the craniosacral motion of the central nervous system.
Lateral	towards one side
Lateral fluctuation	any lateral or circular fluid motion created by the presence of an inertial fulcrum
Life statement	a core belief we have about ourselves and the world
Ligament	a type of connective tissue which connects one bone to another, helping to stabilize a joint
Limbic system	part of the brain which is primarily concerned with autonomic functions, and certain aspects of emotion and behaviour
Longitudinal fluctuation	the motion of fluid and potency along the longitudinal axis of the body. Usually used to describe the inherent motion of cerebrospinal fluid during the cranial rhythmic impulse.
Long tide	the initial and subtlest tidal unfoldment of the Breath of Life which rhythmically moves at about 100 seconds per cycle
Lumbar	relating to the five vertebrae of the lower back just above the sacrum
Lumbosacral junction	the joint between the last lumbar vertebra (L5) and the sacrum
Lymphatic	pertaining to the vessels and the lymph fluid within them which are part of the body's immune system
Lymphocyte	a type of cell carried within the lymphatic system, which helps to fight infection
Lymphokine	a substance released by lymphocytes which helps to activate an immune response. Can also send messages to the central nervous system.
Mandible	the lower jaw bone

Maxillae	paired bones which form the upper jaw, part of the face and the lower part of the orbits
Medial	towards the midline
Meninges	the membranous lining of the central nervous system which is composed of the dura mater, the arachnoid and the pia mater
Meridian	a channel through which vital force or *chi* passes, according to the Chinese medical system
Mesenchym	a matrix of connective tissue, in the middle of the three layers of rudimentary tissues in the embryo
Metopic suture	a suture dividing the left and right parts of the frontal bone, which is present at birth and usually fuses by the age of seven. In about 10 per cent of people it persists throughout life
Midline	the central axis of the body which divides it equally into right and left sides
Mid-tide	the second tidal unfoldment of the Breath of Life, which moves into inhalation and exhalation at about 2.5 cycles per minute. The driving force behind the cranial rhythmic impulse.
Motility	a motion which arises from within a structure – its inner rhythmic pulsation
Moulding	the shaping of a baby's skull bones as a result of forces exerted on it during birth; a treatment approach in which the practitioner encourages the gentle restoration of the normal contours of the skull
Nadi	a channel through which vital force passes around the body, according to the Ayurvedic system of medicine
Nasal bones	paired bones which form part of the arch of the nose
Neural tube	a hollow structure formed in the embryo around which the central nervous system grows
Neuro-transmitter	a chemical substance released by nerve cells and which is used to communicate signals from one nerve cell to another
Neutral	a point at which the forces around an inertial fulcrum have reached a balance (same as point or state of balanced tension). **Practitioner neutral** – a level of attention which is ideal for craniosacral palpation and treatment, where the practitioner's attention is at rest between 'coming and going' and is devoid of expectation or need
Notochord	a rod-shaped cord of cells, formed along the primal midline, defining the axis for embryological development
Nuclei (singular: nucleus)	a group of nerve cells, usually in the central nervous system, which relate to the functioning of a particular nerve
Occipital bone (occiput)	the bone which forms the back and part of the floor of the skull. Contains the foramen magnum.
Oedema	an accumulation of fluid

Olfactory nerve	a cranial nerve which passes through small holes in the ethmoid bone, relaying the sense of smell
Orbit	the bony walls which contain the eye
Original matrix	our blueprint of health; an original intention for health which is never lost
Osteopathic lesion	an osteopathic term to describe a place of restricted motion and impaired function
Osteopathy	a system of health care developed by Dr Andrew Taylor Still which places an emphasis on the relationship between body structure and function, and which views the body as a whole unit which is capable of healing itself when its structure and function are in alignment
Palatine bones	paired bones forming the back portion of the hard palate at the roof of the mouth, part of the walls of the nasal cavity and a small part of the orbit
Palpate	to examine by touch
Palpation	the act of sensing through the hands
Parasympathetic nervous system	the branch of the autonomic nervous system which emerges from the brainstem and the sacral region of the spinal cord. Involved with maintaining the functions of the body in states of rest and relaxation.
Parietal bone	paired bones which form a large part of the posterior roof and sides of the cranium
Pathology	the manifestation of disease; the study of disease processes
Periosteum	a connective tissue covering which closely adheres to the surface of bones
Petrous ridge	an angled ridge along the inside of the temporal bone, providing the attachment for the lateral border of the tentorium cerebelli
Physiology	the study of the way the body functions
Pia mater	innermost layer of the meningeal membrane system, closely adhering to the contours of the central nervous system
Pineal gland	a hormonal gland located at the back wall of the third ventricle, which is involved with sleep and reproduction
Pituitary gland	a small gland which is considered to be the 'master gland' of the hormonal system, sitting in the sella turcica of the sphenoid bone
Placebo	an inactive substance often used in controlled studies to test drugs, but which may nevertheless provide therapeutic benefits
Plexus (plural: plexi)	a network of vessels or nerves
Point of balanced tension	a point at which the tensions of the tissues around an inertial fulcrum have reached an equal and neutral balance. An optimal point for inertia to resolve.
Polarity therapy	a therapeutic system, developed by Dr Randolph Stone, which seeks to balance the constitutional energies of a patient
Posterior	towards the back of the body

Potency	strength, force or power. An intelligent force which maintains order and balance and which is carried in the fluid systems of the body. *Inertial potency* – the concentration of forces which have become bound up at an inertial fulcrum.
Primal midline	the midline orientating force that provides the axis for the growth and development of the embryo, and continues to act as an organizational force for the expression of primary respiratory motion
Primary respiratory mechanism	the core tissues which express primary respiratory motion, consisting of the inherent fluctuation of cerebrospinal fluid, the motility of the central nervous system, the mobility of the intracranial and intraspinal membranes, the mobility of cranial bones and the involuntary motion of the sacrum between the iliac bones of the pelvis
Primary respiratory motion	rhythmic motion produced by the Breath of Life which is expressed as the long tide, the mid-tide and the cranial rhythmic impulse
Primary respiratory system	the whole system of rhythmic motion produced by the Breath of Life, including the long tide, the mid-tide, the cranial rhythmic impulse and the ground of stillness from which these rhythms arise
Psycho-neuro-immunology (P.N.I.)	the study of the physiological relationship and mechanisms of communication between the mind, the nervous system and the immune system
Quantum physics	the study of the smallest units into which matter can be broken down
Reciprocal tension membrane system	the dural membrane system which surrounds and partitions the central nervous system, and which is attached to and continuous with cranial bones and the sacrum. It is relatively inelastic and always held in a state of reciprocal tension during its motion.
Reference beam	a pure beam of laser light which is reflected onto a photographic plate to produce a hologram
Resource	something which supports health and balance
Sacro-iliac	pertaining to the joint between the iliac bone of the pelvis and the sacrum
Sacrum	the bone at the base of the spine located between the ilia, composed of five fused vertebrae
Sagittal suture	the joint between the two parietal bones along the top of the cranium
Secondary respiration	lung breathing
Sella turcica	a concave saddle-shaped notch on the upper surface of the sphenoid bone, in which the pituitary gland sits
Shape	an inertial pattern which has become retained in the tissues
Shock	an event which can overwhelm our ability to respond effectively
Shutdown	a sudden cessation of the cranial rhythmic impulse which occurs with a state of overwhelm

Spheno-basilar junction (S.B.J.)	the joint between the sphenoid bone and the occiput, formed of cartilage which fuses in adulthood, but nevertheless allows for small degrees of motion. Considered to be the natural fulcrum for the craniosacral motion of all other bones in the body.
Sphenoid bone	a bone which forms the front part of the cranial floor, the back part of the orbits and a part of the temples
Sphenopalatine ganglion	a bundle of nerve cells located between the sphenoid and palatine bones, from which branches supply the tear ducts and lining of the nose
Spina bifida	a failure of the vertebral column to close during embryological development, leaving a space through which the spinal cord and membranes may protrude
Spinal accessory nerve	a cranial nerve supplying muscles of the neck and shoulder girdle, exiting from the skull via the jugular foramen
State of balance	a balancing of the forces which control the presence of an inertial fulcrum, accessed via the mid-tide or the long tide. A state of optimal opportunity for the resolution of inertial forces.
Stillpoint	a temporary cessation of primary respiratory motion, marked by a time of deep physiological rest during which the fluids can recharge with potency
Straight sinus	a drainage channel which is formed at the junction between the falx cerebri and the tentorium cerebelli. It is angled posteriorly and inferiorly at about 30 degrees; the location of Sutherland's fulcrum.
Subarachnoid space	the space between the arachnoid and the pia mater, which contains cerebrospinal fluid
Superior	towards the upper part of the body
Sushumna	a channel of energy along the central column of the spine according to yogic practice, the central rod of the caduceus
Sutherland's fulcrum	the natural fulcrum of the reciprocal tension membrane system, located at the straight sinus (formed within the junction between the falx cerebri and the tentorium cerebelli). This fulcrum automatically shifts along the straight sinus during the inhalation and exhalation phases of the cranial rhythmic impulse
Suture	a specialized joint of the bones of the cranium
Sympathetic nervous system	the branch of the autonomic nervous system which originates in the thoracic and lumbar regions of the spinal cord, and which is concerned with body activities in states of stress or activity
Systemic Lupus Erythematosus (SLE)	a connective tissue disorder, related to an impaired function of the immune system
Temporal bone	paired bones which form part of the sides of the skull, containing the organs of hearing and balance

Temporo-mandibular joint (T.M.J.)	the joint between the temporal bone and the mandible, i.e. the jaw joint
Tentorium cerebelli	the part of the reciprocal tension membrane system, formed of dura and shaped like a tent, which provides a horizontal partition between the upper and lower parts of the brain
Thoracic	the middle part of the spine consisting of 12 vertebrae which provide attachment for the ribs; sometimes called 'dorsal'
Thymus gland	a gland located at the centre of the chest which matures lymphocytes, and which is particularly important for the immune functioning of babies and children
Tide	an involuntary rhythmic motion expressed as inhalation and exhalation
Tissue	an aggregation of cells, which are grouped together for a common function
Tissue memory	the imprint of experiences, perhaps containing an emotional or psychological aspect, which are held within tissues
Traction	a movement of two structures away from each other
Transverse	horizontal, side-to-side
Trauma	an event or series of events, created by danger which mobilizes the body's protective mechanisms
Traumatization	the result of being overwhelmed by trauma and not having the resources to dissipate the effects
Trophism	nourishment
Umbilicus	'belly button'. The mark left at the place where the umbilical cord attached a baby to its mother
V-spread	a treatment approach, usually used at sutures or joints, during which fluid and potency are directed towards an inertial fulcrum with one hand, whilst disengagement is facilitated by spreading the two fingers of the other hand
Vagus nerve	a 'wandering' cranial nerve which enters the body and supplies many internal organs, including the throat, heart, lungs and most of the digestive system. These paired nerves form 95 per cent of the parasympathetic nervous system.
Vault	the bones of the upper part of the cranium which are embryologically formed from membrane
Venous sinus	channel which drains cerebrospinal fluid and de-oxygenated blood away from the head. Many venous sinuses are formed within the folds of the cranial dural membranes.
Ventouse	a suction appliance which is used to pull a baby out from the birth canal
Ventricle	a cavity of the brain which contains cerebrospinal fluid
Vertebra	a bone of the spine
Vomer	a thin triangular-shaped bone which is located between the lower surface of the sphenoid bone and the hard palate
Zygomae	paired bones which form the prominences of the cheeks and the lateral walls of the orbit

REFERENCES

REFERENCES

INTRODUCTION

1   In this context, the term 'biodynamic' was coined by Dr Rollin Becker D.O.
2   This idea is found in Indian culture, some Native American traditions and esoteric Judaism.

CHAPTER 1

1   Dr H. Magoun D.O., *Osteopathy in the Cranial Field* (3rd edn; The Sutherland Cranial Teaching Foundation, 1976): xi
2   Dr W. G. Sutherland D.O., *Teachings in the Science of Osteopathy* (Rudra Press, 1991): 4
3   Dr W. G. Sutherland D.O., *Contributions of Thought* (The Sutherland Cranial Teaching Foundation, 1967): 49
4   Professor Giuseppe Sperino, *Anatomia Umana* (vol. 1): 203
5   Hugh Milne, *Heart of Listening* (North Atlantic Books, 1995): 54
6   Emmanuel Swedenborg, *The Cerebrum and Its Parts* (vol. 1 of *The Brain Considered Anatomically, Physiologically and Philosophically*; Swedenborg Scientific Association, 1938): 209
7   Sutherland, *Contributions*: 102–3
8   Dr A. T. Still, *Autobiography of A. T. Still* (A. T. Still; reprinted by the American Academy of Osteopathy, 1981): 235
9   Sutherland, *Contributions*: 102
10   Sutherland, *Science of Osteopathy*: 14
11   Sutherland, *Contributions*: 142
12   N.B. This concept is found in traditional Chinese, Ayurvedic and Tibetan systems of healing and was also referred to by Hippocrates as 'the healing power of nature'.
13   Dr Harold Magoun D.O., *Osteopathy in the Cranial Field* (1st edn; Sutherland Cranial Teaching Foundation, 1951): 15
14   Sutherland, *Contributions*: 97
15   Sutherland, *Contributions*: 138–9
16   Dr John Upledger D.O., *Your Inner Physician and You* (North Atlantic Books, 1991): 15
17   Dr John Upledger D.O., 'Differences Separate CranioSacral Therapy from Cranial Osteopathy', *Massage and Bodywork* Autumn 1995
18   Sutherland, *Science of Osteopathy*: 14
19   Sutherland, *Contributions*: 143

CHAPTER 2

1   Rabindranath Tagore, *Gitanjali* (Macmillan, 1912): 85 (verse 69)

2   Itsuo Tsuda, *The Dialogue of Silence* (trans Giorgia Capra; Luni Editrice Milano, 1992)

3   Dr V. M. Frymann D.O., 'A Study of the Rhythmic Motions of the Living Cranium', *JAOA* 70, May 1971: 928–45. Reprinted in Richard Freely D.O. (ed), *Clinical Cranial Osteopathy* (The Cranial Academy)

4   Melicien Tettambel D.O., Allen Cicora B.S., Edna Lay D.O., F.A.A.O., 'Recording of the Cranial Rhythmic Impulse' (Kirksville College of Osteopathic Medicine). Originally published in *JAOA* 78, October 1978: 149. Reprinted in Richard Freely D.O. (ed), *Clinical Cranial Osteopathy* (The Cranial Academy)

5   Hugh Milne, *The Heart of Listening* (North Atlantic Books, 1995): xviii

6   John E. Upledger and Zvi Karni, 'Mechanical Electric Patterns During Craniosacral Osteopathic Diagnosis and Treatment', *JAOA* 78 (1979): 782–91

7   Z. Karni, J. E. Upledger, J. Mizrahi, L. Heller, E. Becker and T. Najenson, 'Examination of the Cranial Rhythm in Long-Standing Coma and Chronic Neurological Cases', in John Upledger and Jon Vredevoogd, *Craniosacral Therapy* (Eastland Press, 1983): Appendix B

8   Milne, *Heart of Listening*: 4

9   John M. McPartland D.O., M.S. and Eric A. Mein M.D., 'Entrainment and the Cranial Rhythmic Impulse', *Alternative Therapies* 3.1, January 1997

10 Franklyn Sills M.A., R.C.S.T., *Craniosacral Biodynamics* (draft version. North Atlantic Books, 2001)

11 Dr Rollin Becker D.O., *Life in Motion* (Rudra Press, 1997): 124

12 Dr James Jealous D.O., 'Around the Edges', *The Tide* [newsletter of the Sutherland Society, UK] Spring 1996

13 Phrase coined by Franklyn Sills M.A., R.C.S.T.

14 Anecdote from Colin Perrow R.C.S.T.

15 Dr W. G. Sutherland D.O., *Contributions of Thought* (Sutherland Cranial Teaching Foundation, 1967): 39

16 Dr Rollin Becker D.O., *Diagnostic Touch: Its Principles and Application, Part 4: Trauma and Stress* (Academy of Applied Osteopathy, 1965 Yearbook, vol. 2)

17 Dr Michael Shea, *Somatic Cranial Work* (Shea Educational Group, 1997): 61

18 Dr W. G. Sutherland D.O., *Teachings in the Science of Osteopathy* (Rudra Press, 1991): 14

19 Sutherland, *Contributions*: 102

20 Sutherland, *Contributions*: 130

21 Sutherland, *Teachings*: 14

22 *N.B.* Some practitioners also refer to an even slower motion which arises as a kind of wellspring, with each outgoing upsurge arising about every 20–25 minutes. This motion keeps spreading out into space until a new 'tide' arises

23 Genesis 2:7 (King James version)

24 The Buddha, *Prajnaparamita Heart Sutra* (trans Ven. Thich Nhat Hanh, *The Heart of Understanding*; Parallax Press, 1988): 1

25 Sutherland, *Teachings*: 16

26 Ibid.

27 Dr James Jealous D.O., 'Healing and the Natural World', (interview in *Alternative Therapies* 3.1, January 1997)

28 Dr Rollin Becker D.O., *The Stillness of Life* (Stillness Press, 2000): 6

29 Sutherland, *Contributions*: 203

30 'Shape-shifting' is a term used to denote an ability of Native American shamans to change their form.

31 Dr David Bohm, in Ken Wilber (ed), *The Holographic Paradigm* (Shambhala Publications, 1982): 190

32 After Franklyn Sills M.A., R.C.S.T., *The Polarity Process* (Element Books, 1989): 14

33 Sills, *Craniosacral Biodynamics*

34 Wilber, *Holographic Paradigm*: 2

35 Sills, *Craniosacral Biodynamics*

36 Ibid.

37 Dr Karl Pribram, *Languages of the Brain* (NJ: Prentice-Hall, 1971)

38 Wilber, *Holographic Paradigm*: 9

39 'Is it done with mirrors?', *Rhythm and News* Spring 1997. Originally published in Marilyn Ferguson, *Brain/Mind* (Interface Press, 1996)

40 Dr Ray Gottlieb, *Brain/Mind Bulletin* 21.6, March 1996

41 Grahame Whitehead, 'Living Water', *Positive Health* March 2000

42 After Sills *Polarity Process*: 17

43 Ibid.

44 Vera Stanley Alder, *From the Mundane to the Magnificent* (Rider, 1988): 75

45 Henry Lindlahr M.D., *Philosophy of Natural Therapeutics – vol. 1* (Maidstone Osteopathic Clinic, 1975): 24

46 Wilber, *Holographic Paradigm*: 3

47 Jealous, 'Around the Edges'

48 E. Blechschmidt and R. Gasser, *Biokinetics and Biodynamics of Human Differentiation* (Springfield, IL: Charles C. Thomas, 1978): xiii

49 Blechschmidt and Gasser, *Biokinetics and Biodynamics*

50 Sills, *Craniosacral Biodynamics*

51 Jealous, 'Healing and the Natural World'

52 Sills, *Craniosacral Biodynamics*

53 Jealous, 'Around the Edges'

54 Case history from Colin Perrow R.C.S.T.

55   Sutherland, *Science of Osteopathy*: 14

56   Becker, *Life in Motion*: 41

CHAPTER 3

1   Dr Rollin Becker D.O., *Life in Motion* (Rudra Press, 1997): 119

2   Franklyn Sills M.A., R.C.S.T., *Craniosacral Biodynamics* (draft version. North Atlantic Books, 2001)

3   Ibid.

4   Dr W. G. Sutherland D.O., *Teachings in the Science of Osteopathy* (Rudra Press, 1991): 5

5   Becker, *Motion*: 41

6   John Nolte, *The Human Brain* (3rd edn; Mosby, 1993): 59

7   R. F. Erlinghauser, *The Circulation of Cerebrospinal Fluid through the Connective Tissue System* (Academy of Applied Osteopathy Year Book, 1959): 77–87

8   Dr A. T. Still, *Philosophy of Osteopathy* (Kirksville, MO: A. T. Still, 1899): 39

9   Reynold Spector and Conrad Johanson, 'The Mammalian Choroid Plexus' [quoting experiments by Volzhina and Klovosky], *Scientific American* November 1989

10   Ibid.

11   J. Hilton, *Rest and Pain* (Philadelphia: J.B. Lippincott Co., 1950): 25

12   Magoun, *Cranial Field* (3rd edn): 34

13   Dr W. G. Sutherland D.O., *Contributions of Thought* (Sutherland Cranial Teaching Foundation, 1967): 202

14   Dr Rollin Becker D.O., *The Stillness of Life* (Stillness Press, 2000): 5

15   Magoun, *Cranial Field* (3rd edn): 42

16   Dr John Upledger D.O., *The Brain Is Born* (North Atlantic Books, 1996): 333

17   Dr John Upledger D.O. and Jon Vredevoogd, *Craniosacral Therapy* (Eastland Press 1983): 12

18   Still, *Philosophy of Osteopathy*: 39

19   Sutherland, *Science of Osteopathy*: 14

20   Sutherland, *Contributions*: 243

21   Magoun, *Cranial Field* (3rd edn): 25

22   Becker, *Motion*: 90

23   Sutherland, *Contributions*: 140

24   Dr Randolph Stone D.O., *Polarity Therapy – Complete Collected Works, Volume 1* (CRCS Publishers, 1986): 30

25   Sutherland, *Contributions*: 140

26   R. T. Lustig, in Magoun, *Cranial Field* (3rd edn): 26

27   Burton, from 'Anatomy of Melancholy', in Manly Hall, *Man, Grand Symbol of the Mysteries* (The Philosophical Research Society, 1972): 138

28   Hall, *Man, Grand Symbol*: 140–5

29   Magoun, *Cranial Field* (1st edn; 1951): 15

30   See L. C. Clark, 'Discussion of evidence for the participation of serotonin in mental processes' *Annals of the New York Academy of Sciences* Part 3 (March 14th, 1957): 668; H. Hyden, 'Satellite cells in the central nervous system', *Scientific American* 205, December 1961: 62; R. O. Becker, 'Bioelectricity: a new frontier' [report on research at the Veterans Administration Hospital, Syracuse, NY], *Modern Medicine* November 11th 1963: 64

31   D. Feinberg and A. Mark, 'Human brain motion and cerebrospinal fluid circulation demonstrated with MR Velocity imaging', *Radiology* 163 (1987): 793–9

32   A. M. Lassek, *The Human Brain* (C. C. Thomas, 1957)

33   After Upledger, *The Brain is Born*: 53

34   N.B. The axis of rotation for the curling and uncurling of the central nervous system passes through the two Foramina of Monro, the channels which connect the lateral ventricles with the third ventricle

35   Sutherland, *Contributions*: 160

36   Robert Ornstein and David Sobel, *The Healing Brain* (Macmillan 1989): 36

37   Dr A. T. Still, *Autobiography* (Dr A. T. Still, 1897): 219. Quoted in Sutherland, *Contributions*: 239

38   Stanley Keleman, *Emotional Anatomy* (Center Press, 1985): 52

39   Sutherland, *Contributions*: 236

40   Sills, *Craniosacral Biodynamics*

41   Harish Johari, *Chakras: Energy Centres of Transformation* (Rochester, VT: Destiny Books, 1987): 21

42   Magoun, *Cranial Field* (3rd edn): 30

43   Sutherland, *Contributions*: 38

44   Sutherland, *Contributions*: 156

45   Upledger and Vredevoogd *Craniosacral Therapy*: 87

46   N.B. Chi Kung is an ancient Chinese system of exercises to help balance energy flow in the body

47   Don Cohen D.C., *Introduction to Craniosacral Therapy* (North Atlantic Books, 1995): 3

48   Magoun, *Cranial Field* (3rd edn): 32

49   Sutherland, *Contributions*: 138

50   Ibid.

51   Sutherland, *Contributions*: 135

52   Hugh Milne, *Heart of Listening* (North Atlantic Books, 1995): 8

53   N.B. Detailed descriptions of the craniosacral motion of each bone can be found in various textbooks – see, for example, Magoun, *Osteopathy in the Cranial Field*; Upledger and Vredevoogd, *Craniosacral Therapy*; Milne, *The Heart of Listening*, Brookes; *Lectures on Cranial Osteopathy*

54   Dr James Jealous, 'Around the Edges'

55   Sutherland, *Science of Osteopathy*: ix

56   Sutherland, *Contributions*: 230

57   Dr A. T. Still, as quoted in Sutherland, *Science of Osteopathy*: x

58   After Franklyn Sills M.A., R.C.S.T.

59   Sills, *Craniosacral Biodynamics*

60   Erlinghauser, *Circulation of Cerebrospinal Fluid*

61   Claire Dolby D.O., R.C.S.T., *Connective Tissues* (unpublished): 1

62   Erlinghauser, *Circulation of Cerebrospinal Fluid*

63   Still, *Philosophy of Osteopathy*: 162, 164

64   Upledger and Vredevoogd, *Craniosacral Therapy*: 236

65   H. Frohlich, *International Journal of Quantum Chem* 2, 1968: 641–9

66   Dr Will Wilson R.C.S.T., 'The Mystery of Craniosacral Therapy', *The Fulcrum* [Craniosacral Therapy Association, UK] Winter 1998/99

67   Upledger and Vredevoogd, *Craniosacral Therapy*: 236

68   Upledger and Vredevoogd, *Craniosacral Therapy*: 46

69   Keleman, *Emotional Anatomy*: 69. Also see Wilhelm Reich, *Character Analysis* (NY: Farrar, Straus and Giroux, 1949)

70   After Paul Vick R.C.S.T.

71   This analogy has been adapted from an original idea by Dr W. G. Sutherland, *Contributions*: 147, and also Dr Joseph Goodman D.O., N.D.

CHAPTER 4

1   Jelaluddin Rumi, *The Essential Rumi* (trans Coleman Barks with John Moyne; Harper Collins, 1995): 15

2   Dr A. T. Still, *Autobiography of A. T. Still* (A. T. Still, reprinted by American Academy of Osteopathy, 1981): 195

3   Dr James Jealous D.O., 'Healing and the Natural World' (interview in *Alternative Therapies* 3.1, January 1997)

4   *Dorlands Pocket Medical Dictionary* (23rd edn; W. B. Saunders, 1982)

5   Still, *Autobiography*: 282

6   Dr Viola Frymann D.O., *Collected Papers of Viola Frymann* (American Academy of Osteopathy, 1998): 243

7   Frymann, *Collected Papers*: xx

8   Still, *Autobiography*: 32

9   Still, *Autobiography*: 252

10   Carter H. Downing D.O., *Principles and Practice of Osteopathy* (Tamor Pierston, 1981): 18

11   Charles Bowles, D.O., quoted in Dr Rollin Becker D.O., *The Stillness of Life* (Stillness Press, 2000): 254

12   Rev Martin Luther King Jr, *The Ethical Demands for Integration* [12/7/62] and *A Testament of Hope* (James M. Washington, ed; Harper, 1991): 122

13   Elizabeth Hayden D.O., *Osteopathy for Children* (Elizabeth Hayden, Churchdown Osteopaths, 1997): 5

14   Dr I. M. Korr, *The Biological Basis for the Osteopathic Concept* (American Academy of Osteopathy Yearbook 1960: 130; reprinted from the *Journal of Osteopathy* LXI.4, April 1954)

15   Ven. Sogyal Rinpoche, talk in London, 1998

16   N.B. Dr John Upledger uses this term to denote our inner wisdom which can be contacted to provide guidance in the process of treatment, *Your Inner Physician and You* (North Atlantic Books, 1991): 111

17   Still, *Autobiography*: 88

18   Dr W. G. Sutherland D.O., *Contributions of Thought* (Sutherland Cranial Teaching Foundation, 1967): 114

19   Henry Lindlahr M.D., *Philosophy of Natural Therapeutics – vol. 1* (Maidstone Osteopathic Clinic, 1975): 26

20   Dr Rollin Becker D.O., *Life in Motion* (Rudra Press, 1997): 21

21   Becker, *Motion*: 125

22   Lindlahr, *Philosophy*: 19

23   Jealous, 'Healing and the Natural World'

24   Dr James Jealous D.O., 'Around the Edges', *The Tide* [newsletter of the Sutherland Society UK] Spring 1996

25   Dianne M. Connelly, *All Sickness Is Homesickness* (2nd edn; Columbia, MD: Traditional Acupuncture Institute, 1993): 46

26   Hugh Milne, *The Heart of Listening* (North Atlantic Books, 1995): 70, 73

27   Stephanie Hiller, *Stop, Listen, Act* (Brainwave/Holistic London Guide, Summer 1999)

28   Surya Das, *The Snow Lion's Turquoise Mane* (HarperSanFrancisco, 1992): inscription

29   Sutherland, quoted by Dr Rollin Becker in Foreword of *Teachings in the Science of Osteopathy* (Rudra Press, 1991): xii

30   Franklyn Sills M.A., R.C.S.T., *Craniosacral Biodynamics* (draft version. North Atlantic Books, 2001)

CHAPTER 5

1   Dr Rollin Becker D.O., *Life in Motion* (Rudra Press, 1997): 62

2   Becker, *Motion*: 178

3   E. Blechschmidt and R. Gasser, *Biokinetics and Biodynamics of Human Differentiation* (Springfield, IL: Charles C. Thomas, 1978)

4   Franklyn Sills M.A., R.C.S.T., *Lecture on the Tides* (June 1998; unpublished)

5   Katherine Ukleja D.O., R.C.S.T. Personal communication.

6   Dr John Upledger D.O., *The Brain Is Born* (North Atlantic Books, 1996): 363

7   Franklyn Sills M.A., R.C.S.T., *Craniosacral Biodynamics* (Draft version. North Atlantic Books, 2001)

8   Ibid.

9   Dr Rollin Becker D.O., *Diagnostic Touch: Its Principles and Application* (Academy of Applied Osteopathy, 1963 Yearbook)

10   Sills, *Craniosacral Biodynamics*

11   Dr Michael Shea, *Somatic Cranial Work* (Shea Educational Group, 1997): 54

12   Becker, *Diagnostic Touch*

13   Ibid.

14   N.B. The work of Dr William Emerson, one of the world's leading psychologists working in the field of pre-natal trauma, provides much 'anecdotal' evidence of the responsiveness of cells from the very beginnings of life. Also see John Rowan, paper entitled *Major Categories of Early Psychosomatic Traumas*, 1978; Ronald Laing, *Facts of Life* (Penguin, 1976); Nandor Fodor, *In Search of the Beloved* (NY: University Books, 1949)

15   Jelaluddin Rumi, in Andrew Harvey (trans), *Love's Fire* (MOTH)

16   Sills, *Craniosacral Biodynamics*

17   Gabrielle Roth, *Sweat Your Prayers* (Jeremy P. Tarcher, 1997): 4

18   Concept developed by Franklyn Sills M.A., R.C.S.T.

19   Dr W. G. Sutherland D.O., *Contributions of Thought* (Sutherland Cranial Teaching Foundation, 1967): 147

20   Dr James Jealous D.O., 'Healing and the Natural World' [interview by Bonnie Harrigan], *Alternative Therapies* 3.1, January 1997: 68–76

21   S. Suzuki, *Zen Mind, Beginner's Mind* (NY: Weatherhill, 1991)

22   Dr A. T. Still, *Philosophy of Osteopathy* (Kirksville, MO: 1899): 39

23   Ibid.

24   Sutherland, *Contributions*: 85

25   Dr John Upledger D.O. and Jon Vredevoogd, *Craniosacral Therapy* (Eastland Press, 1983): 260

CHAPTER 6

1   Lao Tze, extract from *Tao Te Ching*.

2   Dr James Jealous D.O., 'Healing and the Natural World' [interview by Bonnie Harrigan], *Alternative Therapies* 3.1, January 1997: 68–76

3   Jelaluddin Rumi, *The Essential Rumi* (trans. Coleman Barks with John Moyne; Harper Collins, 1995): 261

4   Wendy Webber, 'Relationships', *London and S.E. Connections* 24, Aug/Nov 1999
5   Franklyn Sills M.A., R.C.S.T., *Craniosacral Biodynamics* (Draft version. North Atlantic Books, 2001)
6   Ibid.
7   Ibid.
8   Dr Rollin Becker D.O., *Life in Motion* (Rudra Press, 1997): 155
9   Dr W. G. Sutherland D.O., *Contributions of Thought* (Sutherland Cranial Teaching Foundation, 1967): 146
10 A. Guggenbuhl-Craig, *Power in the Helping Professions* (NY: Spring Publications, 1971)
11 S Strogatz , I Stewart. 'Coupled oscillators and biological synchronization', *Scientific American* 269.12 (1193): 102–9. Quoted by Leon Chaitow N.D., D.O., 'Integrated Medicine, Cranial Influence – becoming a heavy pendulum?', *Positive Health Magazine* March 1999
12 Chaitow, 'Integrated Medicine, Cranial Influence'
13 Ibid.
14 Instruction from H. H. the 12th Gyalwang Drukpa, head of the Drukpa Kargyud school of Tibetan Buddhism
15 Nelson Mandela, Presidential Inaugural Speech, South Africa 1994
16 Dr Rollin Becker D.O., *Life in Motion* (Rudra Press, 1997): 160
17 Sills, *Craniosacral Biodynamics*
18 Ibid.
19 Diagram based on an original idea by Ged Sumner R.C.S.T.
20 Hugh Milne, *The Heart of Listening* (North Atlantic Books, 1995): 132
21 Don Cohen D.C., *An Introduction to Craniosacral Therapy* (North Atlantic Books, 1995): 68
22 Milne, *The Heart of Listening*: 131
23 Sills, *Craniosacral Biodynamics*
24 Dr John Upledger D.O., *Your Inner Physician and You* (North Atlantic Books, 1991): 99
25 Sills, *Craniosacral Biodynamics*
26 This story was told by Franklyn Sills, M.A., R.C.S.T.
27 Dr Rollin Becker D.O., *Diagnostic Touch: Its Principles And Application, Part 4: Trauma and Stress* (Academy of Applied Osteopathy, 1965 Yearbook, vol 2)
28 S. Suzuki, *Zen Mind, Beginner's Mind* (NY: Weatherhill, 1991)
29 Dianne M. Connelly, *All Sickness Is Homesickness* (Columbia, MD: Traditional Acupuncture Institute, 1993): 98
30 Dr H. Magoun D.O., *Osteopathy in the Cranial Field* (3rd edn; Sutherland Cranial Teaching Foundation, 1976): 81
31 Dr Will Wilson R.C.S.T., 'The Mystery of Craniosacral Therapy', *The Fulcrum* Winter 1998/99
32 Sills, *Craniosacral Biodynamics*
33 Becker, *Diagnostic Touch, Part 1 (1963)*

34   Milne, *The Heart of Listening*: 134

35   Becker, *Diagnostic Touch, Part 1*

36   Dr John Upledger D.O., *Craniosacral Therapy 2, Beyond the Dura* (Eastland Press, 1987): 216

37   Ibid.

38   Becker, *Motion*: 6

39   Upledger, *Craniosacral Therapy 2*: 218

40   Anecdote told by Franklyn Sills M.A., R.C.S.T.

41   This story told by Jack Kornfield, during a talk 'A Path with Heart', London, May 1999

42   W. Heisenberg, *Physics and Philosophy: The Revolution in Modern Science* (Harper, 1958)

43   Dr Rollin Becker D.O., *Diagnostic Touch: Its Principles And Application, Part 2* (Academy of Applied Osteopathy, 1964 Yearbook)

44   Analogy devised by Katherine Ukleja D.O., R.C.S.T.

45   The term *biosphere* was coined by Becker, *Diagnostic Touch: Part 4*

46   From lecture by Katherine Ukleja D.O., R.C.S.T. London, 1999

47   Gabrielle Roth, *Sweat Your Prayers* (Jeremy P. Tarcher/Putnam, 1998): 29

48   Anecdote from Colin Perrow R.C.S.T.

49   Sills, *Craniosacral Biodynamics*

50   Jealous, 'Healing and the Natural World'

51   H. H. the 12th Gyalwang Drukpa, 'Teachings on the Bardo', England 1995. The term *lama* refers to someone who is an accomplished spiritual practitioner.

52   Magoun, *Osteopathy in the Cranial Field*: 81

CHAPTER 7

1   Dr A. T. Still, quoted in Dr Rollin Becker, *Life in Motion* (Rudra Press, 1997): 116

2   Hugh Milne, *The Heart of Listening* (North Atlantic Books, 1995): 2

3   Matthew Appleton R.C.S.T., 'Every Body Tells a Story', *South West Connection* April/July 2000 (Wessex Connections Ltd)

4   Dr W. G. Sutherland D.O., quoted in Dr H. Magoun, *Osteopathy in the Cranial Field* (3rd edn; Sutherland Cranial Teaching Foundation, 1976): 99

5   Dr John Upledger D.O., *Your Inner Physician and You* (North Atlantic Books, 1991): 60

6   Michael Burghley, *The Heart of the Healer* (Aslan Publishing, 1987): 19

7   Franklyn Sills M.A., R.C.S.T., *Craniosacral Biodynamics* (draft version. North Atlantic Books, 2001)

8   Dr H. Magoun, *Osteopathy in the Cranial Field* (3rd edn; Sutherland Cranial Teaching Foundation, 1976): 99

9   Magoun, *Osteopathy in the Cranial Field*: 100

10   Dr Michael Shea, *Somatic Cranial Work* (Shea Educational Group, Inc., 1997): 81

11   Franklyn Sills M.A., R.C.S.T., *Lecture on the Tides* (June 1998; unpublished)

12   Dr James Jealous D.O., 'Healing and the Natural World' [interview by Bonnie Harrigan], *Alternative Therapies* 3.1, January 1997: 68–76

13   Sills, *Lecture on the Tides*

14   Becker, *Motion*: 245

15   Sills, *Craniosacral Biodynamics*

16   Becker, *Motion*: 5

17   Dr Rollin Becker, *Diagnostic Touch: Its Principles and Application, Part 4: Trauma And Stress* (vol. 2; Academy of Applied Osteopathy, 1965 Yearbook)

18   Dr A. T. Still, *Autobiography* (Dr A. T. Still, 1908; reprinted by American Academy of Osteopathy, 1981): 224

19   Becker, *Diagnostic Touch: Its Principles and Application, Part 3* (Academy of Applied Osteopathy, 1964 Yearbook)

20   Ibid.

21   Dr James Jealous D.O., 'Around the Edges', *The Tide* [newsletter of the Sutherland Society UK] Spring 1996

22   Anecdote from Colin Perrow R.C.S.T.

23   Carlos Castaneda, *The Teachings of Don Juan* (Penguin Books, 1976): 182

24   Sills, *Craniosacral Biodynamics*

25   Sills, *Karuna Institute Prospectus*, 1999

26   Sutherland, quoted in Dr Rollin Becker, *Life in Motion* (Rudra Press 1997): 34

27   Sills, *Craniosacral Biodynamics*

28   Dr Rollin Becker, 'The Cerebrospinal Fluid as a Mechanism' *The Cranial Letter* 47.1 (Winter): 6–7

29   Dr Rollin Becker, *The Stillness of Life* (Stillness Press, 2000): 30

30   Adapted from a story told by Ven. Sogyal Rinpoche, London, 1996

31   Dianne M. Connelly, *All Sickness Is Homesickness* (2nd edn; Columbia, MD: Traditional Acupuncture Institute, 1993): 5

32   Becker, *Motion*: 246

33   Dr John Upledger and Jon Vredevoogd, *Craniosacral Therapy* (Eastland Press, 1983): 21

34   Douglas Janssen R.C.S.T., R.P.P., *Training Prospectus* (Watertown, MA: Craniosacral Institute, 2000)

35   Sills, *Craniosacral Biodynamics*

36   Dr W. G. Sutherland D.O., *Contributions of Thought* (Sutherland Cranial Teaching Foundation, 1967): 139

37   Magoun, *Osteopathy in the Cranial Field*: 100

38   Sills, *Lecture on the Tides*

39   Ven. Gyetrul Jigme Rinpoche, 'The Teachings and Practices of King Gesar of Ling' (talk in London, September 1999)

40 Anecdote from Colin Perrow R.C.S.T.

41 Dr Viola Frymann D.O., *Collected Papers of Viola Frymann* (American Academy of Osteopathy, 1998): 68

42 Frymann, *Collected Papers*: 69

43 Sills, *Craniosacral Biodynamics*

44 Magoun, *Osteopathy in the Cranial Field*: 83

45 Magoun, *Osteopathy in the Cranial Field*: 85

46 Upledger, *Your Inner Physician*: 30

47 Magoun, *Osteopathy in the Cranial Field*: 108

48 Dr Will Wilson R.C.S.T., 'The Mystery of Craniosacral Therapy', *The Fulcrum* Winter 1998/99 (Craniosacral Therapy Association, UK)

49 Becker, *Motion*: 28

50 Dr W. G. Sutherland D.O., *Contributions*: 140

51 Sutherland, *Teachings in the Science of Osteopathy* (Rudra Press, 1991): 14

52 Sutherland, *Contributions*: 137

53 T. S. Eliot, extract from 'Burnt Norton' in *Four Quartets* (Faber and Faber, 1986): 15

54 Rollin Becker D.O., 'Using the Stillness', from Scientific Section of *The Cranial Letter: The Teachings of Rollin E. Becker D.O.* 51.2 (May 1998)

55 Sutherland, *Science of Osteopathy*: 16

56 Lao Tzu, *Tao Te Ching*, extract from Stephen Mitchell, *The Enlightened Heart* (Harper and Row, 1989): 14

57 Sutherland, *Contributions*: 137

58 Carol Manheim and Diane Lavett, *Craniosacral Therapy and Somato-Emotional Release* (SLACK Inc., 1989): 17

59 Sills, *Craniosacral Biodynamics*

60 Katherine Ukleja D.O., R.C.S.T./Claire Dolby D.O., R.C.S.T., training course notes

61 R. Smoley, 'Exploring Craniosacral Therapy', *Yoga Journal* May/June 1991: 20–4

62 Carol Manheim and Diane Lavett, *Craniosacral Therapy and Somato-Emotional Release* (SLACK Inc., 1989): 83

63 After Franklyn Sills M.A., R.C.S.T. *The Polarity Process* (Element Books, 1989): 135

64 Ambrose and Olga Worrall, *The Gift of Healing* (Harper and Row, 1965): 123

65 Becker, *Stillness*: 2

66 Magoun, *Osteopathy in the Cranial Field*: 105

67 Carlisle Holland D.O., J. H. Holland, 'Perceptual transference, a scientific basis for intuition and other paranormal experiences' (unpublished manuscript); quoted in Shea, *Somatic Cranial Work*: 33

68 Becker, *Stillness*: 10

69 Hermann Hesse, *Magister Ludi, The Glass Bead Game* (Bantam Books, 1980)

CHAPTER 8

1   Tsong Khapa, in Thubten Jigme Norbu and Colin Turnbull, *Tibet, Its History, Religion and People* (Penguin/Pelican, 1972)

2   H. R. H. Prince Charles, quote from a speech given to the British Medical Association on 14th December 1982

3   Mij Ferrett R.C.S.T., 'Retrieving Innocence via Experience', *Caduceus* 33, Autumn 1996

4   The term *energy cyst* was coined by Dr John Upledger D.O.

5   Franklyn Sills M.A., R.C.S.T., *Craniosacral Biodynamics* (draft version. North Atlantic Books, 2001)

6   Dr John Upledger D.O., *Craniosacral Therapy 2, Beyond the Dura* (Eastland Press, 1987): 213

7   Linda Lazarides, *Principles of Nutritional Therapy* (Thorsons, 1996): 61, 90; Elizabeth Lipski M.S., C.C.N., *Digestive Wellness* (2nd edn; Keats Publishing, 2000): 100

8   Dr James Jealous D.O., 'Around the Edges', *The Tide* [newsletter of the Sutherland Society, UK] Spring 1996

9   Sills, *Craniosacral Biodynamics*

10   H. H. the 14th Dalai Lama, London, May 1999

11   The Buddha, extract from the *Dhammapada*

12   Ken Dychtwald, *Bodymind* (Jeremy P. Tarcher, 1986): 22

13   Ron Kurtz and Hector Prestera, *The Body Reveals* (Harper and Row, 1976): 1

14   Ibid.

15   Marilyn Ferguson, in Ken Dychtwald, *Bodymind* (Jeremy P. Tarcher, 1986): Foreword

16   Albert Vorspan, *I'm OK, You're a Pain in the Neck* (Doubleday and Co., 1976): 21

17   Endorphins are the type of neuro-transmitter which carry out this function.

18   The famous experiments by Pavlov showed how the physiological responses of dogs could be conditioned. A bell was rung just before the dogs were fed and, after a short while, the dogs would automatically salivate just at the sound of the bell.

19   Dr Robert Ader and Dr Nicholas Cohen, 'Behavioural Reconditioned Immunosupression', *Psychosomatic Medicine* 37 (1975): 333–40

20   Ida Rolf, 'Structural Integration', *Systematics* 1.1 (June 1963): 9–10

21   Dr John Upledger D.O. and Jon Vredevoogd, *Craniosacral Therapy* (Eastland Press, 1983): 141

22   Dr Viola Frymann D.O., *Collected Papers of Viola Frymann* (American Academy of Osteopathy, 1998): 250

23   Dr Wilhelm Reich, in Dr Ken Dychtwald, *Bodymind* (Jeremy P. Tarcher, 1986): 102–3

24   Dychtwald, *Bodymind*: 103

25   For the American reader, this means 'a complete screw-up'

26   Kurtz and Prestera, *The Body Reveals*: 3

27   Dychtwald, *Bodymind*: 14

28   Robert Fulford D.O., *Dr Fulford's Touch of Life* (Pocket Books, 1997): 29

29   Frymann, *Collected Papers*: xix

30   Hollis Pecora and Paul Benson, *Noni News #5* (Devon: Resonance, 1999)

31   Franklyn Sills M.A., R.C.S.T., *Lecture on the Tides* (June 1998; unpublished)

32   Frymann, *Collected Papers*: 317

33   Jocelyn Proby D.O., in Henry Lindlahr, *Philosophy of Natural Therapeutics* (Maidstone Osteopathic Clinic, 1975): 3

34   Harold Saxton Burr, *Blueprint for Immortality* (Neville Spearman, 1972)

35   Franklyn Sills M.A., R.C.S.T., *The Polarity Process* (Element, 1989): 47

36   Dr Randolph Stone D.O., *Polarity Therapy – Complete Collected Works* (C.R.C.S. Publishers, 1986): 30

37   Sills, *Craniosacral Biodynamics*

38   Sills, *Polarity Process*: 45

39   Dr Elmer Green, in Upledger and Vredevoogd, *Craniosacral Therapy* (Eastland Press, 1983): xii

40   N.B. Many sources describe seven chakras, including a crown chakra at the top of the head. However, in the Ayurvedic and Tibetan tradition this seventh chakra is not considered to be a 'true' chakra, as it is only activated when all the others are fully open

41   Dr Viola Frymann D.O., 'The Law of Mind, Matter and Motion – Scott Memorial Lecture', *Yearbook of the American Academy of Osteopathy* 73 (1973): 13–22

42   Ibid.

43   Frymann, *Collected Papers*: xix

44   Becker, *Stillness of Life*: 2

45   Albert Einstein, in Caroline Latham, *The Heart of Healing* (Findhorn Press, 2000): 15

46   Albert Einstein, in Becker, *Stillness of Life*: 255

CHAPTER 9

1   Ernest Hemingway, *A Farewell to Arms*

2   Penguin Medical Encyclopaedia *(Penguin, 1972)*

3   *Concise Oxford English Dictionary* (7th edn; Oxford University Press, 1982)

4   Dr Peter Levine, *Waking the Tiger* (North Atlantic Books, 1997)

5   Levine, *Waking the Tiger*: 155

6   Dr Hans Selye, *The Stress of Life* (NY: McGraw-Hill, 1956)

7   Levine, *Waking the Tiger*: 19

8   Lecture by Scott Zamurut R.C.S.T., Boston, MA, 1999

9   Levine, *Waking the Tiger*: 20

10   Levine, *Waking the Tiger*: 149

11   J. Axelrod and T. D. Reisine, 'Stress Hormones, Their Interaction and Regulation', *Science* 224

(1984): 452–9. Quoted in Bessel van der Kolk M.D., *The Body Keeps the Score: Memory and the Evolving Psychobiology of Post-traumatic Stress* (Harvard Medical School, 1994)

12   Levine, *Waking the Tiger*: 32

13   Axelrod and Reisine, 'Stress Hormones'

14   Sigmund Freud, *Introduction to Psychoanalysis and the War Neurosis* (Standard edn; J. Strachey [trans and ed]; Hogarth Press, 1919/1954): 17:207–10

15   Dr Rollin Becker D.O., *The Stillness of Life* (Stillness Press, 2000): 45

16   Dr A. T. Still, *Autobiography of A. T. Still* (A. T. Still, reprinted by American Academy of Osteopathy, 1981): 88

17   Norman Cousins, *Anatomy of an Illness* (Bantam, 1984)

18   Research quoted in Daniel Goleman and Joel Gurin (eds), *Mind Body Medicine* (Consumer Reports Books, 1993)

19   Dr James Jealous D.O., 'Accepting the Death of Osteopathy: A New Beginning', (Thomas Northrup Lecture, reprinted in *AAO Journal*, Winter 1999)

20   Dr Rollin Becker, *Life in Motion* (Rudra Press, 1997): 247

21   Arthur Janov, *The Primal Scream* (Abacus, 1973)

22   Dr Rollin Becker D.O., *Diagnostic Touch: Its Principles and Application, Part 4, Trauma and Stress* (Academy of Applied Osteopathy, 1965 Yearbook)

23   Levine, *Waking the Tiger*: 10

24   Franklyn Sills M.A., R.C.S.T., *Craniosacral Biodynamics* (Draft version. North Atlantic Books, 2001)

25   H. H. the 14th Dalai Lama, London, May 1999

26   Eugine Gendlin, *Focusing* (Bantam Books, 1981)

27   Franklyn Sills M.A., R.C.S.T., *Focusing Notes* (unpublished)

28   Levine, *Waking the Tiger*: 12

29   Levine, *Waking the Tiger*: 187

CHAPTER 10

1   Ella Wheeler Wilcox, in Beryl Arbuckle D.O., *The Dynamics of Cerebrospinal Fluid* (American Academy of Osteopathy Yearbook, 1950; reprinted in *Selected Writings of Beryl Arbuckle*; PA: National Osteopathic Institute and Cerebral Palsy Foundation, 1977): 97

2   Haven Trevino, *The Tao of Healing* (New World Library, 1999)

3   Elizabeth C. Hayden D.O., *Osteopathy for Children* (Elizabeth Hayden, Churchdown Osteopaths, 1997): 3

4   Dr Viola Frymann D.O., 'Relation of Disturbance of Craniosacral Mechanism to Symptomatology of the Newborn: Study of 1,250 Infants', in *The Collected Papers of of Viola Frymann* (American Academy of Osteopathy, 1998): 8

5   Frederick Leboyer, *Birth without Violence* (Mandarin Paperbacks, 1991): 23

6   M. Lietaert Peerbolte, *Psychic Energy in Prenatal Dynamics* (Wassenaar, The Netherlands: Service Publishers, 1975)

7   Dr John Upledger D.O., *The Brain Is Born* (North Atlantic Books, 1996): 30

8   Dianne M. Connelly, *All Sickness Is Homesickness* (Columbia, MD: Traditional Acupuncture Institute, 1993): 25

9   John Rowan, paper entitled *Major Categories of Early Psychosomatic Traumas*, 1978

10   Ronald Laing, *Facts of Life* (Penguin, London, 1976)

11   Nandor Fodor, *In Search of the Beloved* (NY: University Books, 1949)

12   Maura Sills, lecture notes on *Core Process Psychotherapy*

13   Ibid.

14   Ibid.

15   Dr William Emerson Ph.D., *Infant and Child Birth Re-facilitation*, transcription of presentation to Second International Congress on Pre- and Perinatal Psychology, San Diego, CA, 1985

16   Ibid.

17   Dr William Emerson Ph.D., personal lecture notes

18   Upledger, *The Brain Is Born*: 35

19   Dr William Emerson Ph.D., personal lecture notes

20   Gordon Bourne, *Pregnancy* (Pan Books, London, 1975): 66

21   Upledger, *The Brain Is Born*: 38

22   Upledger, *The Brain Is Born*: 40

23   Franklyn Sills, M.A., R.C.S.T., personal lecture notes

24   Jonathan Curtis Lake D.O., from an article and talk entitled *The Sum of the Parts*. Unpublished

25   Ibid.

26   Hayden, *Osteopathy for Children*: 3

27   Hayden, *Osteopathy for Children*: 10

28   Gerard Tortora and Nicholas Anognostakos, *Principles of Anatomy and Physiology* (4th edn; Harper and Row, 1984): 723

29   Janet Balaskas and Dr Yehudi Gordon, *The Encyclopedia of Pregnancy and Birth* (Little, Brown and Company, 1998)

30   Hayden, *Osteopathy for Children*: 16

31   Frymann, *Collected Papers*: 3

32   Hayden, *Osteopathy for Children*: 27

33   Arbuckle, *Selected Writings*: 81

34   Dr Ray Castellino D.C., R.P.P. and Debby Takikawa D.C., 'Delivery Self-attachment and Bonding – Part 2', *The Fulcrum* Autumn 1999

35   Robert Fulford D.O., *Dr Fulford's Touch of Life* (Pocket Books, 1997)

36   Fulford, *Touch of Life* (quoting studies by Dr Bertil Jacobsen at the Karolensha Institute, Sweden)

37   Dr Ken Dychtwald, *Bodymind* (Jeremy P. Tarcher, 1986): 33

38   Janet Balaskas, *New Active Birth* (Thorsons, 1989): 140

39   Balaskas and Gordon, *Encyclopedia*: 164

40   Balaskas and Gordon, *Encyclopedia*: 146

41   Leboyer, *Birth without Violence*: 70

42   Leboyer, *Birth without Violence*: 64

43   Castellino and Takikawa, *The Fulcrum*, Autumn 1999

44   Hayden, *Osteopathy for Children*: 8

45   Lennart Righard M.D. and Margaret Alade R.N., *Delivery Self-Attachment* (1990): 1106–7

46   Castellino and Takikawa, *The Fulcrum*, Autumn 1999

47   Righard and Alade, *Delivery Self-Attachment*: 1106–7

48   Dr A. G. Cathie, *Growth and Nutrition of the Body with Special Reference to the Head* (Academy of Applied Osteopathy Yearbook 1962): 149–53

49   Steve Jones *et al.*, *The Cambridge Encyclopedia of Human Evolution* (Cambridge University Press, 1994): 108

50   Upledger, *The Brain Is Born*: 289

51   Ibid.

52   Dr John Upledger D.O. and Jon Vredevoogd, *Craniosacral Therapy* (Eastland Press, 1983): 263

53   Dr H. Magoun D.O., *Osteopathy in the Cranial Field* (3rd edn; Sutherland Cranial Teaching Foundation, 1976): 101

54   Leboyer, *Birth without Violence*: 42

FURTHER READING

BOOKS ON CRANIOSACRAL THERAPY
AND CRANIAL OSTEOPATHY

Franklyn Sills M.A., R.C.S.T., *Craniosacral Biodynamics* (North Atlantic Books, 2001)

Rollin Becker D.O., *Life in Motion: The Osteopathic Vision of Rollin E. Becker* (Stillness Press, 1997)

—, *The Stillness of Life* (Stillness Press, 2000)

W. G. Sutherland D.O., *Contributions of Thought* (2nd edn; Sutherland Cranial Teaching Foundation, 1998)

—, *Teachings in the Science of Osteopathy* (Anne Wales, ed.; Sutherland Cranial Teaching Foundation, 2000)

H. I. Magoun D.O., *Osteopathy in the Cranial Field* (1st edn 1951, 3rd edn 1976; Sutherland Cranial Teaching Foundation)

A. T. Still, *Autobiography of A. T. Still* (A. T. Still 1908; reprinted by the American Academy of Osteopathy, 1981)

Viola Frymann D.O., *The Collected Papers of Viola Frymann* (American Academy of Osteopathy, 1998)

Michael Shea, *Somatic Cranial Work* (Shea Educational Group Inc., 1997)

John Upledger and Jon Vredevoogd, *Craniosacral Therapy* (Seattle: Eastland Press, 1983)

John Upledger, *Craniosacral Therapy II, Beyond the Dura* (Seattle: Eastland Press, 1987)

—, *Your Inner Physician and You* (North Atlantic Books, 1991)

—, *Somato-Emotional Release and Beyond* (North Atlantic Books, 1992)

—, *A Brain Is Born* (North Atlantic Books, 1996)

Hugh Milne, *The Heart of Listening Volumes 1 & 2* (North Atlantic Books, 1998)

Beryl Arbuckle D.O., F.A.A.O., *The Selected Writings of Beryl Arbuckle* (PA: National Osteopathic Institute and Cerebral Palsy Foundation, 1977)

Elizabeth Hayden D.O., *Osteopathy for Children* (Elizabeth Hayden, Churchdown Osteopaths, 1997)

Dennis Brookes, *Lectures on Cranial Osteopathy* (Thorsons, 1981)

Robert Fulford D.O., *Dr Fulford's Touch of Life* (Pocket Books, 1997)

RELATED SUBJECTS

Peter A. Levine, *Waking the Tiger* (North Atlantic Books, 1997)

Ken Wilber (ed.), *The Holographic Paradigm* (Shambhala, 1982)

Ken Dychtwald, *Bodymind* (Jeremy Tarcher Inc, 1986)

Ron Kurtz and Hector Prestera, *The Body Reveals* (Harper & Row, 1976)

Stanley Keleman, *Emotional Anatomy* (Center Press, 1985)

Henry Lindlahr, *Philosophy of Natural Therapeutics Volume 1* (Maidstone Osteopathic Clinic, 1975)

Franklyn Sills, *The Polarity Process* (Element Books, 1989)

Dianne M. Connelly, *All Sickness Is Homesickness* (Columbia, MD: Traditional Acupuncture Institute, 1993)

Gabrielle Roth, *Sweat Your Prayers* (Jeremy P. Tarcher/Putnam, 1998)

Dawson Church and Alan Sher (eds), *The Heart of the Healer* (NY and Mickleton: Aslan Publishing 1987)

Tom Dummer D.O., *Tibetan Medicine* (Routledge, 1988)

Deane Juhan, *Job's Body, A Handbook for Bodyworkers* (Station Hill, 1995)

Robert Ornstein and David Sobel, *The Healing Brain* (Papermac/Macmillan, 1989)

Hans Selye, *The Stress of Life* (McGraw-Hill, 1956)

Eugine Gendlin, *Focusing* (Bantam, 1981)

Keith Moore and T. V. N. Persaud, *Before We Are Born* (W. B. Saunders, 1998)

Frederic Leboyer, *Birth Without Violence* (Mandarin Paperbacks, 1991)

David Chamberlain, *The Mind of Your Newborn Baby* (North Atlantic Books, 1998)

RESOURCE GUIDE

FINDING A THERAPIST

Registers of Practitioners

An asterisk (*) indicates the main registers of practitioners trained in a biodynamic model of craniosacral work

UK

* Craniosacral Therapy Association
Monomark House
Old Gloucester Street
London WC1N 3XX
Tel: 07000 784735
email: info@craniosacral.co.uk
website: http://www.craniosacral.co.uk

International Cranial Association
478 Baker Street
Enfield
Middlesex EN1 3QS
Tel: 0208 367 5561
email: kbs07@dial.pipex.com

Craniosacral Society
2 Marshall Place
Perth PH2 8AH
Tel: 01738 629444
Fax: 01738 442275
email: mail@craniosacral.org

Sutherland Cranial College
(osteopaths only)
Spring Vale
Mill Hill
Brockweir
Gloucester NP6 7NW
Tel/fax: 01291 689908
email: suthcranialcoll@compuserve.com

USA and Canada

* Craniosacral Therapy Association of North America (C.S.T.N.A.)
1110 Birchmont Road
Unit 21
Scarborough
Ontario M1K 1S7
Tel: (416) 755 7734
Fax: (416) 755 9771
email: info@craniosacraltherapy.org
website: www.craniosacraltherapy.org

American Craniosacral Therapy Association
11211 Prosperity Farms Road
Suite D-325
Palm Beach Gardens, FL
33410-3487
Tel: (561) 622 4334
email: upledger@upledger.com

Sutherland Cranial Teaching Foundation
(osteopaths, medical doctors, dentists)
4116 Hartwood Drive
Fort Worth, TX
76109
Tel/fax: (817) 926 7705

The Cranial Academy
(osteopaths, medical doctors, dentists)
8202 Clearvista Parkway
Suite 9-D
Indianapolis, IN
46256
Tel: (317) 594 0411
Fax: (317) 594 9299

Switzerland

* Schweizerischer Berufsverband für Craniosacral-Therapie (SBCT)
Postfach
CH-8044 Zurich
Tel: 0878 800 214
Fax: 041 320 8530
email: info@cranioverband.ch

Schweiz. Dachverband für Craniosacral-Therapie
Lindenweg 10
CH-4414 Fullinsdorf BL
Tel: 61-9039503
Fax: 61-9039501
email: contact@sdvc.ch

Spain

* Asociacion Espanola De Terapia Craneosacral
Apartado 391
08800 Vilanova i la Geltru
Tel: 93-743 2455 or 93-815 8163

Training Schools

UK
An asterisk (*) denotes courses accredited by the Craniosacral Therapy Association UK

* Craniosacral Therapy Educational Trust
78 York Street
London W1H 1DP
Tel/fax: 07000 785 778
email: info@cranio.co.uk
website: www.cranio.co.uk

* Karuna Institute

Natsworthy Manor
Widecombe-in-the-Moor
Newton Abbot
Devon TQ13 7TR
Tel/fax: 01647 221457
email: karuna@eurobell.co.uk

* College of Craniosacral Therapy

9 St Georges Mews
London NW1 8XE
Tel: 0207 483 0120

International Cranial Association

478 Baker Street
Enfield
Middlesex EN1 3QS
Tel: 0208 367 5561
email: kbs07@dial.pipex.com

Sutherland Cranial College

(open to osteopaths only)
Spring Vale
Mill Hill
Brockweir
Gloucester NP6 7NW
Tel/fax: 01291 689908
email: suthcranialcoll@compuserve.com

Upledger Institute

2 Marshall Place
Perth PH2 8AH
Tel: 01738 444404
Fax: 01738 442275
email: mail@upledger.co.uk

USA

An asterisk (*) denotes courses accredited by the Craniosacral Therapy Association of North America

* Craniosacral Institute (Boston and Chicago)
17 Spring Street
Watertown, MA
02472
Tel: (617) 924 9150 or 800 875 6347
Fax: (617) 924 2828
email: energydj@aol.com
website: www.americanschoolforenergytherapies.com

* Shea Educational Group Inc.
13878 Oleander Avenue
Juno Beach, FL
33408-1626
Tel: 1-800-717 7432
email: sheagroup@aol.com

* Polarity Center Colorado
1721 Redwood Avenue
Boulder, CO
80304
Tel: (303) 443 9847
website: www.PolarityColorado.com

* Lifeshapes
39582 Via Temprano
Murrieta, CA
92563
Tel: (909) 607 0652

* Institute of Complementary Therapies
758 Kapahulu Avenue
Unit 501
Honolulu, HI
96816
Tel: (808) 734 5272

Sutherland Cranial Teaching Foundation

(open to osteopaths, medical doctors and dentists)
4116 Hartwood Drive
Fort Worth, TX
76109
Tel/fax: (817) 926 7705

The Cranial Academy

(open to osteopaths, medical doctors and dentists)
8202 Clearvista Parkway
Suite 9-D
Indianapolis, IN
46256
Tel: (317) 594 0411
Fax: (317) 594 9299

Upledger Institute Inc.

1211 Prosperity Farms Road
Suite D-325
Palm Beach Gardens, FL
33410-3487
Tel: (561) 622 4334
email: upledger@upledger.com

Canada

An asterisk (*) denotes courses accredited by the Craniosacral Therapy Association of North America

* Institute of Complementary Therapies

9251-8 Yonge Street
Unit 245
Richmond Hill
Ontario L4C 9T3
Tel: (416) 879 6702
email: ICTeducate@aol.com

Switzerland

Institut für Ganzheitliche Energiearbeit
Austrasse 38
CH-8045 Zurich
Tel: 01-4616601

Kientalerhof
Centre for Wellbeing and Creativity
CH-3723 Kiental
Tel: 033-6762676
Fax: 033-6761241
email: info@imi-kiental.ch

Spain

Instituto De Terapia Craneosacral
Calle Calvet, 31, 30, 20
Barcelona 08021
Tel: 93-201 4665
email: jfeil1@compuserve.com

European School of Craniosacral Therapy
The Paracelsus Centre
Aptdo. de Correos 554
Javea 03730
Alicante
Tel: 96-5794343
email: rmharris@ctv.es

Germany

Tanmayo Krebber-Woehrle
Adalbertstr. 98
D-80799 Muenchen
Tel: 89-2734 9749
Fax: 89-2734 9748
email: k-woe@t-online.de

Italy

ITCS
Via Litoranea 76
04010 Borgo Sabotino
Latina
Tel/fax: 0773-648283
email: info@craniosacrale.it

New Zealand

Mana Retreat Centre
Coromandel RD1
Tel: 7-866 8972
Fax: 7-866 8214
email: manaretreat@compuserve.com

INDEX